The Knotty Truth

Managing Tightly Coiled Hair at Home

M. Michele George

Manifest Publishing Enterprises, LLC   Columbus, Ohio

The Knotty Truth: Managing Tightly Coiled Hair At Home

ISBN Number
978-0-578-01413-5
0-578014130

2nd Edition

George, M. Michele.
Book Cover & Design by Storme Gray (*www.congobrava.com*)

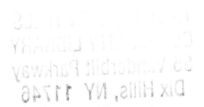

WHAT PEOPLE ARE SAYING ABOUT
THE KNOTTY TRUTH

The Knotty Truth is one of those works that transports the reader from the writer's journey directly into her own. Women of all ages, in all stages of the natural journey and ones who have not yet begun their own will thoroughly enjoy reading this book. As I read, I was transported to different stages of my own life experiences and realized again that all of us have stories to tell and wisdom to impart. Having struggled with the concept of natural hair in America and internationally and conversed with hundreds of women about their hair and identity struggles, I have found that creative and informational resources such as The Knotty Truth are like gold. Through these works, we realize we are not alone in our journeys, our thoughts and feelings. I thoroughly enjoyed The Knotty Truth and I recommend it as a thoughtful, deeply moving and valuable read—full of truth, practical advice and a touch of whimsy in just the right places. Enjoy! **-Patricia Gaines, Executive Founder, Nappturality.com**

I made the dramatic switch from chemical to natural after a series of traumatic experiences. When I started reading The Knotty Truth I did not want to put it down!!!!!! It is a refreshing and revolutionary book that inspired me to not only keep my natural locks, but it has also better prepared me to teach my lovely daughter about what is beautiful about her hair. **-Lena Arnold, Author, <u>For this Child We Prayed: Living with the Secret Shame of Infertility</u>**

A must-read for any woman considering becoming and/or in the midst of being chemical-free. With Knotty Truth, you are armed with information to free yourself; without it, you are like a ship without a sail. As a television personality, this book has added to my confidence to free my mind and escape the chemical! **-Cynthia Barnes Booker, Two-Time Emmy Award Winning Television Anchor/Reporter**

Knotty Note

At the time of writing and publishing the book, I am not a licensed cosmetologist. I am a former customer who grew tired of depending upon the services of an industry that breeds dependence upon chemicals. What I share, I have learned from an online community of women who have successfully grown their hair by breaking away from the traditions taught in beauty schools. I do not dispel the importance of a trained Cosmetolgist-I only mean to offer options to those who do want to learn to care for their hair on their own. My suggestions are not a substitute for the knowledge of a trained cosmetologist; but, rather options that avail themselves if you are willing to learn from others that have found a key to restore their time, money and hair health in their own kitchen.

M. George

SPECIAL THANKS

My husband — you were my personal cheering section of praise and encouragement. Thank you for doing what you do best, I love you.

My sons — you believed I was an author before I did, giving me the push to get this baby into the world. Thanks guys!

My natural family —this project would not have happened without my virtual sisters who stepped in and filled the gap. Because you provided your tips, thoughts, photos, tutorials and more, you made the journey a little bit better for the next sister.

Special thanks to the following ladies for their contributions. I also want to thank the ladies who preferred to remain anonymous to the world; yet, making their mark with their contribution. This project is a collaborative effort birthed out of my sincere desire and their passion to impact more women to join our ever growing community as we embrace the napp, because bad hair is what's good!

Todra Payne, *Celebrity Makeup Artist*
Storme or CongoBrava
Zahara
Corporate Napps
Tiffany
Malaikablu

Yekinae
Gilda
Michelle or Natitwists
Lina
Lady Libra
Sandra
Zulgeil S.

I also want to thank the ladies who preferred to remain anonymous to the world; yet, made their mark on it with their contribution.

Table of Contents

I AM DETERMINED

Where do I get my determination from? I get it from Massa

Who told me I was stupid.
Who told me I was incompetent
Who stripped me of my clothes
Then stripped me of my dignity

Massa' who called me "nappy, uncomely wench" who requires me
to assault my hair equivalent to the assault he took upon my body
in the slave quarters, or wherever he chose to take it.

My body is no longer subject to his assaults; but my hair is.
As I subject it to meet unattainable standards of beauty reserved
for women without a pattern to their hair,
and unable to naturally defy the affects of gravity.

I am determined to master my hair and no longer willing to subject
my temple to harmful chemicals that would unclog bathroom
drains and straighten my hair all in one shot.

I am determined to grow, open and learn the infinite possibilities
that are beholden to God's Queens of the Earth: made from the
Rib of man: made from Earth.

I am determined to challenge the establishment that wants me to
reject what is beholden to God: my crown. And I will wear it with
all the pride, dignity and courage that was denied my ancestors.

Because NOW I am determined.

MGeorge, 2008

10

MY JOURNEY

in search of the nappy headed girl
that was born with hair like Jesus

God gives us all we need

My mind was not settled. It felt betrayed. There's nothing worse than looking in the mirror and not liking what you see. Where can you hide?

My view of beauty was limited and in my small world, there was only one sister transitioning out of her chemical relaxer. She was six months natural ahead of me and because she stayed true to her "natural journey" she eventually inspired me. Her process wasn't physically attractive to me at first. Unlike her, I broke down and chemically relaxed my hair – going back to 'The Lye.' When I relapsed back to the crack that called, seduced, and courted me, she was the only one not enamored with my long, straight flowing hair.

When she asked, my excuse for relaxing my hair was lame. My desire was to have a "professional hairstyle" for job interviews. Her retort was a list of all the style possibilities I could have pursued. I didn't know what she was talking about. It made me mad that I didn't know what to do with my natural head of hair. I decided to educate myself on the care of my hair. I felt embarrassed that I didn't truly love and accept who God made me to be. This raised personal issues for me. Just how much did I really love God if I sat in judgment of His work?

When I transitioned in 2004, I knew I had to make a decision fast or the creamy crack would call out my name again. My two textures would eventually reach a point of discontent once more if I didn't disconnect the processed hair from my chemical free hair. My two textures didn't like the same products and predictably would become unmanageable. I had to break the communication between the chemical free strands and the chemically processed hair. I had to find help.

My DNA demanded "God wouldn't give it to you if He didn't give you the tools to know what to do!" My Bible said: "Everything God made is good." My mind said: "Well, why is my hair bad?" I pursued wisdom. I courted knowledge. A voice reminded me that once upon a time, my mama did my hair, and she knew what to do. Her mama did her hair and she knew what to do. Her mama did her daughter's hair; and, she knew what to do. So, perhaps, I would inherently know too. This time I would launch out on my journey armed with information. I would find freedom from hairdressers and chemicals. I quit the chemicals and let my hair grow.

I sought help on the Internet and found a sisterhood of women who would come to support, educate and love on me. Dee Coiley (aka Patricia Gaines) followed her passion to expose more women to this chemical free phenomenon and she created http://www.nappturality.com/. Because of this support system, I finally made a successful transition and cut my chemically straightened hair in January 2005. I began my mental transition by reconditioning my view of tightly coiled hair — I plastered pictures of beautiful women with natural hair anywhere and everywhere around me.

With courage I cut off the processed hair. Total panic was upon me; my natural hair was a mangy bush that I did not recognize. I was in shock that my 'stretched' four inches of hair shriveled into maybe an inch and a half after shrinkage. Shrinkage left me feeling naked, defense-less and exposed. In addition, the ends of my hair did not 'curl' into pretty ringlets like I had seen in different online photo albums. Instead, it did this Seventies throw back thing and I looked like a pimp with a bad Jheri curl. A curl that was dying for a fresh application of chemicals and a rod set. I didn't know what the heck I was going to do with it!

My mind and my hair had been in bondage to chemicals, societal perceptions, and an industry that thrived upon my misinformation and preyed upon my ignorance and low self esteem. I decided the cycle would end with me as I released even more information on the care of tightly coiled hair.

This book is a manifestation of my passion; I desire to make it and keep it personal. This is not a Bible on hair care, but a resource that can start you exploring, learning and growing in the care of tightly coiled loose hair. So, pull out your coffee cup and have a sit down. It's you and I; it's time to get schooled in a class that was never offered in your traditional institutions of learning.

Sincerely,

Knotty Note

Why do African American women straighten the naps as soon as they show? Is it because they tell the story of Massa' and the other stories on 'the row'? Do they tell a story of sweat blood and tears that toiled in the cotton fields under the Southern sun that beat down in the heat of the day? Is it because we are afraid to be strong like our mothers who came before? The mothers who survived the rapes, survived babies sold off the plantation, survived her wedded husband being bred like a mule with the other slave hands? In shame we have been taught by generations of mothers to hide our story, as if nobody knows. In ignorance, we hide our naps behind weaves and a wig, pretending it is ours. We believe that because we have the receipt others should buy into it too. We hide our locks of courage because we are ignorant to its power.

M. George

CHAPTER ONE

THE KNOTTY TRUTH

For centuries, tightly curled hair has been labeled: kinky, coon, even bad hair. I too once looked upon my hair as hard to deal with, nappy and unsightly. I am compelled to share my revelations learned through trials and tribulations with a full head of tightly coiled, kinky, thick hair void of chemicals and 110% mine! The resources available on the maintenance and care of naturally tight curly hair expands daily as more women tap into the well of knowledge. It is my hope that my contribution from an emotional vantage point of becoming and remaining 'napptural' will help others adjust and accept all the kinks, coils and textures patterned just for them.

1

HAIR HISTORY

Just how did we get to the point where an image of long silky hair blowing in the wind is our image of beauty? We never had that until we became inbred with another race. The seed of shame, assault of identity, and birth of insecurity and anxiety about naps was never before seen as a point of shame until introduced to Europeans who could not understand it. African hair once represented relationships, status, hierarchy, tribal affiliations, culture and custom. Adornment, style and hair care were meticulously carved into the head as plaits, braids, locks, and coils which gave meaning and purpose to one's place in the African community. When Africans were colonized into slavery, the meaning of our hair care and culture was stripped into submission.

As slaves, newly Americanized Africans were busy surviving everyday life. Hair care products and tools were impractical at best when long, grueling days on the plantation evolved into sharecropping for hundreds of years. The campaign began when Africans arrived in ports across Europe with matted hair full of nits and bugs. After months in the hull of a ship locked in chains, we were greeted with ghastly exclamations of disdain and horror because of our unkempt, matted hair. Once colonized, head coverings were encouraged to conceal what we could not care for. We lacked tools, time and moisture products, from the motherland of Africa.

Then, with 'liberation' from slavery after 1865, the traveling sideshows theatrically preyed upon the anxieties of whites and blacks by displaying distasteful nappy images; thus creating a need for their balms made of propane, kerosene and other harmful chemicals. They promised to transform naps into flowing, straight hair. As a bonus, these traveling minstrels offered magic creams that would bleach the skin white, transforming blacks into white people with beautiful flowing hair that lay flat!

Hair care did not become important until the early 20th Century as it was viewed for the first time as a potential lucrative commodity. The traveling conjure man could package hair concoctions in a jar and prey upon the insecurities of nappy-haired people. It began in the early 1900's with Malone and Madam Walker's hair straightening systems, and then progressed to the potato and lye concoctions of the Jazz era. The Ultra Sheen system of the 50's for men, then later women, and our present day rendition of straightening system dominated with Sodium Hydroxide Lye. We, present day negroes, have also bought into the creative marketing of the minstrel shows: black skin is ugly, dirty and kinky hair is bad. African American women continue to dish out millions of dollars to support these marketing stories, reinforcing to our sons and daughters that being black is not good enough: Our blackness needs to be minimized and altered for acceptance with chemical reapplication every twelve weeks.

Today, the brainwashing continues as we straighten our hair thinking it will make us more acceptable to others. We have passed these ideals on to our daughters who repeat the cycle as a means to survive and succeed in America. So much so, that I've met quite a few white people who think our babies are born with straight hair! Generations of little black girls have grown up in a historical vacuum that is reinforced today by mothers, grandmothers, and the hair care industry. What others frown upon, shun and fear, we have adapted and accepted as our own standard of beauty, instead of embracing the beauty originally given to us.

3

Knotty Note

First, they stripped me of my name. Then, they stripped away my history. They took my God and replaced Him with Them. Now, all I want is to know who I am. Who am I without a name? Who am I without a history? Who am I outside of them? Who am I without them? I don't know. So, I begin with my hair. My hair whispers ancient secrets that empower me. My hair is the only thing that I have that they do not control—all of the spirals, kinks and curls. It is all I have that tells me who I am IN HIM.

MGeorge, 2008

Today, marketing is creative and cunning. The marketers have convinced us that we need a system or kit to tame our hair. We are used behind the scenes in marketing departments to remind other African Americans that only those women with long, flowing straight hair will catch a man's attention. The marketing ploys remind women that we don't know what to do with our crown of hair: "Help me, Dr Miracle, fix this nappy mess!" This message is reinforced with commentators like Imus who feel comfortable screaming phrases of disrespect...."They some nappy headed ho's" referring to the championship Rutgers University Women's Basketball Team. Yet, that message and other media messages prick the minds of all women, those with obvious tightly coiled hair and the less obvious, hidden behind a chemical relaxer or straightening comb. Whether chemically treated or chemically free, these messages hurt us all equally. Eventually, the marketing tactics that assault ethnic features continue to create new consumers with new insecurities.

We also see images on television that reinforce what is acceptable and what is ugly. In music videos the women who have flowing hair with incredible sheen are paraded across the screen. On the contrary, commercials usually show cleaning women with hair in its natural state, tightly curled. As a result, many African American women subconsciously believe that we must also relax our hair for employment and acceptance in America. It is the beauty industry that has created a marketing machine driven off of the insecurities of African American women. A marketing monster that reinforces and reaffirms the rationale that African American women must denature and destroy the chemical bonds in our hair to make it straight and beautiful.

My mother, who came of age in the seventies, reminded me that she had to perm her 'fro to get a job. "The man" was not going to hire any Angela Davis militant Negroes at the bank, grocery store or anywhere else in the Seventies. I respect the walls and barriers she and others had to circumvent to pave a way for their daughters. The sad truth remains however, we continue to teach this concept in a new century that is run by globalization, a world point of view, a very different economy and a new set of rules. This new century is sadly governed by the same perspective of the post civil rights era. Ayana Byrd and Lori Tharp enlighten readers in their book <u>Hair Story: Untangling the Roots of Black Hair in America</u> as they explore the history, pride and shame associated with tightly coiled hair originating out of Africa.

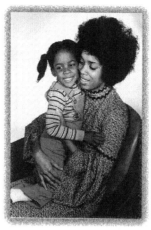

5

These messages impact our psyche from the cradle to the grave. Most little girls want to be loved and accepted more than anything. They grow into women who have the same need if not greater! This example is played out in studies of racial preferences among preschool girls. If an African American girl is given the option of a white or a brown doll, overwhelmingly, she will not choose herself, the brown doll. We can also see this played out at the toy stores — dolls usually left on shelves are brown.

Dr. Kenneth Clark first performed the doll test in 1947. His study helped to desegregate schools in the historic Brown versus Board of Education Case. Almost 55 years later in 2001, Kiri Davis a high school student reenacted the doll test and revealed that our daughters still prefer the white baby to the brown one. Her classmates continued to hold misconceptions of themselves as they wrestled with the same standard that light skinned, "good" haired girls are prettier. This test and many personal testimonies can be viewed on You Tube by using the search words: doll, nappy, or test.

The reality is that we cannot expect our daughters to love and embrace themselves while we alter our skin and our hair with chemicals that mask our own insecurities. Our daughters pick up on this and mirror what they learn. It's one thing to leave their hair natural and, another to see mommy go to the hairdresser and get her hair altered. After all, children do as we do, not as we say. This observed behavior changes to unconscious, learned behavior as we migrate into adulthood, without a conscious thought about it.

6

The brainwashing reinforces and teaches self-hatred, as the beauty industry is a billion dollar industry and growing. All of these mixed signals cause women with tightly coiled hair to question the new growth that bursts through the tiny holes lining our scalps. Hair that refuses to lie down, but reaches in the air generating naturally curly hair that refuses to yield length as a sign of its glory. Hair that produces continual growth which reaches to the sky; hair that defies gravity with strands clinging to one another and banding together in unison. It's a

Knotty Note

I hear God clearer now. I am closer to Him. My antennae is open and the reception is clear. I no longer reject who I am IN HIM. He is pleased. I see him smiling on me now, as I accept His wonderful works through my tresses.

MGeorge, 2008

beautiful thing that leaves many to marvel and despise simultaneously.

We often forget our history and the strength behind our hair, because the texture of tightly coiled hair stirs up controversy now, as it did then. From the basketball courts to the halls of Congress, our texture is a caldron of controversy.

Because of the successful marketing campaign launched against the napp, masses of women with tightly coiled hair get relaxers. As a result, according to the U.S. Bureau of Labor and Statistics, over 600 trained beauticians a year are armed with scissors, clips and chemicals. Perhaps, if we evaluate the client, hair stylist, industry perspective, we will see the driving source of revenue for beauticians. For a beautician to continue to get paid, it is necessary to create a dependency on services: a chemical dependency. If the beautician is not paid, the industry is not paid to produce chemicals. It's a cycle propelled by the consumer: the bottom feeder. Yet, the industry seldom respects its number one customer. We are the consumers who turn our Washington's, Jackson's and Lincoln's over to straight-haired Koreans and no one is giving us a slice of that pie!

According to Aron Ranen's Documentaries on Black Hair Care, featured on You Tube, the Koreans control 80% of the distribution of African American products. The other 20% goes to the white owned companies that provide chemicals to straighten the tightly coiled hair. We must become conscious consumers.

With the wealth of information on the Internet, in print, and organizations rising to address these issues, we can receive and demand the care we deserve. We can support the beauty of tightly coiled hair without conflicting messages. An organization doing something about these inequities is BOBSA; The Black Owned Beauty Supply Association has formed and is addressing this disparity. They exist to raise awareness and empower us by increasing our buying and selling power for beauty supply products. We must support beauty supply stores that are black owned and organizations that are making a stand for us. It doesn't make sense to continuously turn over our money to an industry that doesn't respect the brown behind the green.

Our silence empowers an industry founded upon our vanity. The industry needs tightly coiled girls and women to survive. An industry that puts the distributors, owners and licensors in the suburbs, nice car, phat crib, good schools, while we don't even possess a quarter of their wealth; yet, we steadily hand over our dollars. Quite simply, we need to take back our power, demand good service, and empower ourselves. (It takes effort and we are worth it!)

8

9

One / The Knotty Truth

CHAPTER TWO

CHEMICAL STRAIGHTENING:
why we do it to ourselves

Oppressed hair puts a ceiling on the brain.
- Maya Angelou

Natural hair became my passion when I realized that after almost 40 years on this earth, I did not know how to deal with the lot God gave me. I became determined to style and love my hair as I admired the waves that peeked out between my relaxer touch ups. But to take this journey back to natural required that I process my 'why.' In my mid thirties I began to feel emotions of love and acceptance that I never felt towards my hair before.

For example, to effectively market a product, the motivating factor must be a compelling, resounding 'why.' My why challenged me: "Why do you apply chemicals to your head?" My answer: "For acceptance." I became angrier, "Acceptance from whom? People who really didn't accept my hips, my lips, my skin or the kink of my hair? A people that will take those very attributes off of my body, glue it theirs and call it fashionable and sexy; but, on me ugly?" I wondered why I have to alter myself to fit into a world that will never embrace me anyway. In defiance, I stopped relaxing my hair. I was scared to death; yet, proud of my life decision and became anxious to see where my boldness would take me.

Chemical free since January 2005, I am not some natural vigilante who chooses to scream "Conspiracy!" at the sightings of a chemical. Some chemicals serve decent purposes. Yet, in the case of chemical relaxers, it's difficult for me not to keep the industry's dirty little secret: By design, chemical relaxers strip the hair of vital nutrients, leaving behind a cycle of damaged, dry, and malnourished hair with questionable side effects. The industry would be the last to fund research that proves the harmful effects of chemicals in African American women.

THE RELATIONSHIP BETWEEN HAIR STRANDS AND CHEMICALS

Each hair strand has an outer layer called the cuticle which is the protective sealant of each hair fiber. During the relaxer process the cuticle is removed. The stripping process is necessary to straighten the hair — to access the curly bonds, which lie inside the core of the hair strand. The next layer is the cortex. Underneath, is a nutrient-depleted medulla where the proteins reside and are released from the chemical process.

11

When a chemical relaxer is applied, the cuticle has to be stripped to access the curl bonds, inside this medulla. The curl bonds are straightened and capped when the hair is chemically relaxed straight to prevent coiling. This process of stripping the hair and capping the curly bonds is the only way to make tightly coiled hair elongate. Once the chemical is applied, the tightly coiled hair is permanently altered and cannot be corrected. Because of this alteration, relaxed hair is dry by nature and must be replenished constantly. When this protective cuticle is removed, along with nutrients, the result is a naked, straight hair strand. The cuticles on tightly coiled hair are porous. This causes the hair to react to moisture like a sponge and dry out quickly.

The chemical relaxing process compromises the hair strand, follicles and the scalp condition. As a result, hair once thick may thin or develop bald spots over time; this process is called *Traumatic Alopecia*. African American women suffer from traumatic Alopecia at an alarming rate according to Herbert P. Goodheart, MD (1999). Unfortunately, we take this damage for granted and usually ignore it. The two types of *Traumatic Alopecia* are Scarring and Traction. Scarring Alopecia occurs from inflammation caused by chemicals in the form of hair pomades used during hair straightening with a hot comb or from chemical relaxers.

In *Scarring Alopecia*, the chemical seeps into the hair shaft, impacting the hair follicle which becomes inflamed, exudes puss or may itch. The result is a scab on the scalp after a touch-up. Scabs can form when there's been damage at the follicular level. That's why hairdressers ask if you have been scratching your scalp! If you have scratched, you will have scabs.

12

The follicles are susceptible to damage. Scarring can lead to hair loss permanently or temporary. Hair loss becomes a game of Russian roulette: maybe your hair will grow back, maybe it will become weak and shed over time from breakage or maybe it will not grow back at all. The only thing certain is there will be irregular breakage at the contact point of chemical or heat application on the hair.

Traction Alopecia occurs as a result of tension caused from tight braids or wigs, coarse hair tools or other hairstyles. The first signs of Traction Alopecia are thinning hair edges from the hairline and breakage towards the ears. I experienced this form of alopecia. After years of trying to circumvent it, the only success I had was to leave the chemicals out of my head! Once again, the result can be permanent or temporary and it can result in Scarring Alopecia as well.

For most women, we notice a gradual degradation in the health of our hair. If the wrong type of damage occurs at this level, it is quite possible to experience permanent hair loss. The first signs of chemical or traction alopecia usually show at the temples and crown/ central area of the head. With alopecia from traction, chemicals or straightening, it's difficult to escape these forms of alopecia albeit permanent or temporary. Many women experience thinning, poor quality hair as they age from these disorders. The hair follicles have been worn from years of chemical application. The result is hair loss and hair damage.

Because many women can suffer from a combination of different forms of alopecia, make sure to consult with a licensed dermatologist experienced in scalp disorders to determine if your hair loss is indeed chemical, hormonal or some other form of alopecia. The dermatologist will examine the clinical appearance of your hair, its history and perhaps take a scalp biopsy to examine the follicles. If it is chemically induced damage, there are essential oils (Chapter 4) that can stimulate follicular growth. Protective style choices will also allow the hair to heal and regenerate, if the damage isn't permanent. Finding a hairstyle that minimizes manipulation and product use is the key to regenerating a healthy head of hair.

STRAIGHTENING SYSTEMS

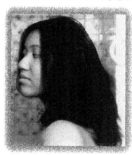
Straightening systems function by stripping the outer cuticle, breaking the curly bonds and capping them. Most Chemical relaxers employ a type of chemical: natural or synthetic, lye or no-lye. They all function to strip the outer cuticle, break the curly bonds and cap them,

compromising the hair. Most chemical relaxers are made from Sodium Hydroxide, but there are other forms.

Temporary Straighteners

Temporary straighteners include tools that are used to style the hair (gas or electric heated devices such as blow driers, curling irons, flat irons, and the hot comb). The hair is straightened with the styling tool and a pomade or heat protectant. The bonds in the hair are temporarily altered to produce a smooth, straight look. The effect of heat is temporary. Over time, the bonds can be hydrated, returning to their original form, like when it rains or water touches the hair.

Sodium Hydroxide/Lye

Sodium Hydroxide (may also come in the form of Sodium Bromide) is the strongest of the chemicals and best known as the one and only original LYE chemical relaxer. Lye relaxers are notorious for their high alkaline content (pH range of 10-14), which is damaging to the hair. Hair strands prefer a neutral pH of 5-6. The high pH factor causes the hair to straighten faster and is caustic in nature. The higher the strength of Sodium Hydroxide, the more corrosive it is to whatever it is applied to (the skin, hair, drain pipe, or oven enamel). When a no-lye Sodium Hydroxide relaxer is used, it simply means that it is man-made, or synthetic, and is marketed as less damaging, while it functions the same as the 'natural' chemical form.

Guanidine Hydroxide/Calcium Hydroxide

Guanidine Hydroxide and Calcium Hydroxide are 'no-lye' relaxers. They are not *harmless* — but *less harmful* than Sodium Hydroxide 'lye' relaxers. It damages the hair also, and requires a neutralizing solution post relaxer application, to stop the straightening process. The same

14

precautions should be taken when applying this chemical to the scalp.

Ammonium Thioglycolate (aka the Jheri Curl)

Ammonium Thioglycolate alters the curl pattern of the hair. Instead of the hair strand lying straight, it has a slight bend, appearing moist, silky, and shiny with loose 'manageable' curls. This chemical is less damaging than the others, but must be complemented with activator juice to replenish lost nutrients during the stripping process.

HAIR COLORING

Commercialized permanent hair colors can damage the hair because the cuticle must be raised to deposit color into the cortex. To lighten the natural color, hair is usually bleached taking melanin or color out, as the new color is deposited into the hair. As a result, the stripping process for coloring can also be damaging and drying. The deposit process can be harmful, as well. When color is deposited, the hair shaft may swell leaving the hair even more susceptible to dryness.

Henna is a form of coloring the hair. Henna is a chemical free, temporary hair color and deep conditioner that can be applied weekly without fear of damage! Complement the use of Henna with a deep setting, **moisturizing** conditioner to balance the Henna and protein molecules. Mixed with egg or olive oil, to enhance and condition the hair at the same time giving it sheen. The conditioning properties of Henna can last for weeks.

Because I am a proponent of natural hair regimes, I encourage Henna over the other hair coloring methods. Henna is a plant protein. Since it's not a chemical, it can be applied often without fear of overlapping. Henna is beneficial for many reasons including the fact that it

15

is free of silicones, it loosens the curl and it is safe for pregnant and nursing mothers. The use of Henna has been known to cure/prevent many scalp conditions such as psoriasis. Henna has even been known to kill head lice and ringworm! Before considering Henna, it's important to test your sensitivity to the plant, to avoid an unnecessary severe allergic reaction. Applying a test sample to inside of the arm may be enough. Be aware that Henna coats, it is a protein and must be supplemented with a moisturizing conditioner.

If the hair is chemically processed, it can be damaging to go from a chemical permanent dye to Henna. So don't do it! (See www.Henna.com for more information on the different types of Henna and how to apply). The Henna website as well as Tulani Kinard's book No Lye is an excellent resource to have when exploring your natural hair care options from coloring to styling. Just apply the directions to good common sense. If the directions say to use gloves, protect the eyes, don't ingest, don't inhale etc...apply this same logic to your use of the chemical on your body. Be conscious, question and seek knowledge. If the hairstylist uses gloves to protect his or her hands, but applies only a coating of Vaseline to *your* scalp—take heed! The stylist's skin is protected from the caustic chemicals, as should you be.

Hair coloring is fun and a simple way to alter your appearance. If you experience a problem contact the FDA and report your reaction: Contact FDA's Center for Food Safety and Applied Nutrition (CFSAN) Adverse Events Reporting System (CAERS): 1-800-FDA-1088 or CAERS@ cfsan.fda.gov.

16

Two / Chemical Straightening

A year ago I stood in the bathtub after I washed my "hair in transition" for the last time. As I looked at the newly emerging curls from my roots fighting to be free it was then, at that moment without any further hesitation, I decided I'm finally ready to chop off the lye...When it was all over, I looked at the 8 inches and years of hair fraud in the garbage. I was free and I was scared. Stunned and kinda shocked as I looked at the Natural me in the mirror, I couldn't even begin to imagine how this journey was going to affect me the way that it has this past year...

-Zhara

CHAPTER THREE

TRANSITION OF THE MIND AND HAIR:
the bend of our hair

TWISTED THINKING

It's easy to make excuses *not* to go natural. Many of us have been taught to hate coiled hair. We learn to hate it before we ever learned to care for it. We were taught that nappy is "African" and we are "American not African." We may have been taught that being "dark and nappy" were two things no one ever would want, or that we had to get along with others and never make them uncomfortable by expressing our curls. What thoughts have gone through your mind?

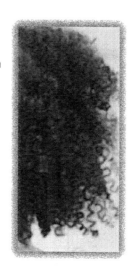

19

- "I have coarse hair."
- "My kitchen is nappy."
- "I don't have that good hair. My hair is a nappy mess."
- "My wooly hair will cut you."
- "I got that African hair."
- "My kitchen is a brillo pad."
- "Natural hair don't look good on everybody, my head is too big."
- "I don't want to be a nappy-headed ho."

For some reason we assume that people may think

we're a Black Panther about to start a revolution if
we are sporting tightly coiled hair! And, we may have
been taught not to remind others of the guilt of slavery,
oppression and suffering — nappy hair does all these
things and more. Nappy hair reminds others what their
hair can't and won't do without enhancements.

As little girls, we watched mama go off to her monthly
hair appointment. We learned how *hard-headed* or *tender-
headed* we were during our daily grooming sessions.
These grooming sessions may have innocuously conveyed
negative perceptions of our kink, linking it by experience
to a source of pain, inability to control, comb and style.
The sessions were accompanied by bows, barrettes,
ponytail holders, combs, brushes, and blue pomade hair
grease. Many little girls learned about the power of Afro
Sheen and it's many uses to straighten, tease and shellac
the hair. Then, sooner than later, many of us are seduced
by the creamy crack of a relaxer.

On the Nappturality.com forum one member shared that
her first chemical relaxer application was at age two!
Another member saw a one year old at the store, with a
relaxer in her head! The mama thought her baby was so
cute, and the baby's edges were already almost burned
out. The psychological damage we have incurred over
our quest to conform is deep. So deeply ingrained in
our minds that this mama hid her baby's napps during
a crucial developmental stage was more important
than allowing the child to develop naturally. Another
member shared that her friend chemically relaxed her
three-year old daughter's hair so it would be pretty
and manageable. Now, the three year old is getting
complements and swinging her hair and mama is sooooo
proud!

These children, like many of us, will never have a conscious memory of self-acceptance and pride. This is the real tragedy. Just how does a person transition away from chemicals when there is no conscious record of chemical-free hair? As a result, so many women grow into a false sense of maturity without the option or the privilege to love themselves the way they were born.

I transitioned in my mid-thirties, while in corporate America. At this time I began to transition my hair and my mind away from chemical dependency. With no more chemical relaxers applied to my scalp, the cloud lifted and I walked in confidence, love and acceptance for me. This awakening has blessed my whole life and I weep for our lost years shrouded in banal ignorance of the power of our tresses.

THE MENTAL JOURNEY

One of the greatest challenges transitioning from chemically relaxed to natural hair is the mental transition. The mental journey is about self-acceptance and learning to care for your hair. Surrounding yourself with a network of brothers and sisters who can pour words of encouragement and support into your journey is key. The physical transition will occur with time; however, a successful mental transition must be deliberate. The mental transition is not a passive event, be diligent. To successfully transition, the mind must be exposed, retrained, reconditioned, open and flexible. A healthy mind is one that is ready to witness the physical transformation of silky hair that 'lyes' straight to kinky hair that defies gravity. Appreciation will come with confidence, sacrifice and focus. Boost your confidence by posting inspiring pictures of hairstyles in the car, your weekly planner, the walls in your bedroom, kitchen, office or the bathroom.

How do you transition in confidence? In order to transition successfully, it is important to understand *how* to transition. It helps to mentally transition when the hair is kept loose and available for experimentation versus bound in braids or twist extensions. However, many do successfully transition with braids and twists catching up on the techniques and nuances of 'doing' the hair later. Regardless of the path, your confidence will grow with your hair, because experimentation leads to interaction with others and the do's and don'ts of hairstyling. Through trial and error and eventually compliments, the confidence will blossom. With proper products and education, you can learn how to style your hair beautifully, even as the texture changes from year to year.

Your transition requires sacrificing vanity and selfish practices that damage hair for the good of healthy growing hair free of chemicals. While building confidence and a network of support, it's critical to remain focused on *your* 'why.' Remember, the 'why' is *your* motivating factor. It is *your* reason for going natural to get you through the rough days when your hair won't act or do right. It's important to remain focused on your why to make it through the rough days, when your hair is only 2-4 inches growing upwardly, instead of downwardly, like it used to. Regardless of the challenges, stay focused. If the goal is hair down the back, stay focused. Every centimeter, inch, foot and yard will grow from the follicle up until a length is reached that weighs your hair down. Focusing and accepting the unique traits of tightly coiled hair will lead to an appreciation of our hair and the depths it will reach with time and self-acceptance.

As often as hairstyles change, the mental transition continues to evolve. When I grew up in the 1980's, the women who wore "naturals" were usually middle-aged women going through menopause wearing teeny weenie afro's (TWAs). Because 'the change' was so severe and uncomfortable, it led to unpredictable hot flashes. Many sweat their hair out so badly that they just cut their hair off and found comfort sporting mini afros. And others who wore dreadlocks were often Rastafarians. I identified with neither group, so it wasn't a consideration for me to go natural until later.

Today, more women are wearing their tightly coiled hair choosing to remain or become natural because of self love, cultural pride, familial pride, spiritual or philosophical reasons. Some simply chose natural hair because it is less maintenance than relaxed hair. These women choose to wear hair free of chemicals because outside approval is no longer required. What a peace there is to look in the mirror and say: "I like what I'm working with!" When we reach this peaceful place it is often lonely and requires courage. Courage that translates into self-confidence can be infectious.

23

I was introduced to chemical relaxers in 1985, at sixteen. My experience mirrors that of many of my sisters who walk in the cloud and have unconsciously been taught to hate their natural hair. Back in the day, getting our hair pressed was like a rite of passage. My monthly washing sessions were traumatic as mama washed through a mat of hair that retained water. After the washes, my hair was knotted up in china bumps section by section in preparation for the hot comb to come hours later after my hair dried. And, oh, the hot comb, that was the worst! Getting my hair pressed was a ritual of smoke, stinky burnt hair, ultra sheen everywhere, the hot comb slipping, promptings to be still from Mama and burns followed with Vaseline and cocoa butter to cover the open wound. The testament of the ordeal was the burned skin (that later turned into a nasty scab of puss, yuck!) on an ear or two when mama pressed the edges.

I longed for the day when I could pass over into the 'nevah nevah' land of ease like my mama and get my hair chemically relaxed. I wanted to be done with all the pain. I concluded that the only way for my dark self to be lovely (with long, flowing hair that blew in the wind) was to have hair like Bo Derek and Farah Fawcett. Becoming Dark 'n Lovely® meant that I would disappear to a quarterly appointment with the hairdresser and get the white paste put on my hair to take away all off my painful kinks and naps. Getting a Dark 'n Lovely® meant I was a woman!

24 Dark 'n Lovely® sealed my fate and that of many others in my generation. A cycle of dependency began: chemical relaxer, hair breakage, trims, braids to give my hair a rest from the damage and grow healthy hair until I relaxed and repeated the cycle again. Once I decided to break free of chemicals in my hair, my mental journey lasted 2.5 years; the mental and physical acceptance was very difficult for me as my hair grew 'up' and not down. It took time to undo a lifetime of negative conditioning towards my hair. But transitioning slowly and trimming away the relaxer helped me to transition mentally and physically, one centimeter at a time.

I too had to venture away from the European standard of beauty seared into my mind. Once my relaxer was completely cut, I felt exposed and hid behind false hair that helped me cope with the changes and allowed me to experience my mental and physical growth. It was my way of transitioning my mind's eye to see my true self. I went through my trials of wigs, pieces, and extension wigs as I dealt with my mental journey, as I learned what worked and didn't work on the weekends. I didn't have a bad hair day because the false hair saved me! I protected my hair under the piece with twists or braids, moisturized and protected by a wig cap. Then, I blended my hair into the false hair.

When I wore the hair through the week, I would always give it a rest and liberate my tendrils on the weekend, letting my curls explode as an offering to the sky. My church was a source of encouragement, because there were many naturals there. On Saturday, it was all about the kids and the family, so it was easy for me to wear my hair out. But, along came Monday, I had to develop a strategy, because I was facing my corporate job, with conservative customers who did not look like me. So, on went the fake hair on Mondays as I tucked away the kinks, curls and naps until Friday. I did this for a year and a half, while I experimented, purchased, practiced and applied new products and tools to my hair.

As my confidence slowly built, I gained the courage to wear my own hair in various styles. The false hair prevented me from being me, and I just couldn't wear it anymore. I couldn't stand my fake self and I strutted my natural hair proudly. When my mental transition caught up with my physical transformation, I had a funeral for my false hair, said good-bye to the Korean hair store and embraced me.

THE PHYSICAL JOURNEY
The physical side of the journey is just as rewarding and adventurous as the mental side. The physical journey is affected by hair textures (tightly coiled, loose, wavy and all textures in between), environments, and genetics. Tightly coiled hair mats, knots, tangles, shrinks and frizzes at will. One head of hair can have more than one

texture on it, making the natural process and lifestyle challenging. The care and maintenance of these different textures can impact the outcome of hairstyles, so it's important to know how to treat them. For example, the warm, humid weather of sunny South Florida is wonderful for tightly coiled hair which soaks up heat and moisture. On the contrary, a dry and arid climate can slow hair growth, exposing it to extreme dryness and damage. Dry indoor heat and dry cool outside air can wreak havoc on moisture retention in the hair, making it dry, brittle and prone to breakage. Learning which products compliment your hair texture and environment in and out of season is critical.

Lifestyles also impact the physical health of the hair. A healthy lifestyle with plenty of fluid intake, exercise, balanced meals and low stress complement good hair growth, sheen and shine. Replenish your body with an adequate supply of water because it keeps the body hydrated on the inside and outside. Exercises that involve inverted positions such as Yoga will help to further stimulate the hair follicles, bringing much needed nutrients, through the blood, to the scalp, aiding in circulation and hair health. Many ladies want to ignore this aspect of hair health; but, it is essential if the hair is to be strong, stay strong and manifest great hairstyles!

Genetics also impact hair growth and health. Your parent's genes are important to take into consideration. Fathers pass the balding gene to daughters and unfortunately, there's nothing that can be done to prevent thinning and balding without intervention. Genetically predisposed, these women should become especially proactive about their hair care and prevent the stress on follicles by eliminating the use of chemicals on the hair. Chemical straightening and hot comb straightening with petroleum-based hair pomade will

26

damage the scalp over time.

The other biological trait affecting the wave of the curly hair is the follicle. There are 3 types of hair follicles: round, oval and oval with a hook. Round follicles produce straight hair that naturally lies flat, seen in Caucasians, Asians and others with straight hair. Flat/ oval follicles with a slight hook (small flap of skin that causes hair to curve) are said to have a 'hook' right below the skin surface at the hair's point of emersion from the scalp, creating the tightly coiled hair. People of African descent will manifest this type of hair. Oval follicles without the hook produce wavy hair that grows out in a wavy formation with a loose curl formation found in mixed populations.

Shrinkage and texture are unique physical characteristics of tightly coiled hair and it can make going natural intimidating. Understanding and embracing tightly coiled hair's purpose can transform and free the transitioning mind! Shrinkage was designed to protect the brain from the sweltering sub-Saharan heat that radiates from the motherland of Africa. It is awesome to think that God loved us enough, that He made the first human with protection and covering!

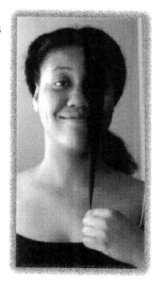

Embracing the bend of the hair and its spongy quality will make your journey easier. Shrinkage occurs when there is water in the air or on the hair, causing the coils to shrink and reduce in length. It can be very frustrating and challenging to deal with shrinkage as it reduces length of ten inches down to anywhere from two to eight inches, depending upon the nature of the curl pattern. Shrinkage occurs, tightly coiled hair primarily grows upwards if it's a tight curl pattern, outwards if it's a looser curl pattern and down if it's wavy. Because tightly coiled hair defies gravity and grows up, humidity can turn the hair into an Afro. (I wish I could count the number of times I would try and pat my hair to lie down, nope, wouldn't do it.)

There are hairstyles and products that can be implemented to define your curl and reduce frizz in the hairstyle chapter. These specific styles compliment a hairstyle that holds relatively well under humid conditions. Because of the nature of the curly bonds, the spring of the curl can condense and loosen. The more moisture in the air, the more tightly compact the hair. The less moisture in the air, the more apt the hair is to stay in a looser curl pattern. Just as melanin captures the sunrays and protects our skin from the dangerous UV radiation, tightly coiled hair functions to protect, giving natural shade.

28

Knotty Note

On the Nappturality forum, it was discussed how women who 'play' in their hair the first year after releasing the chemical, report that they feel more empowered, versus women who continue to have their hair done by stylists or in braids and twists. Do It Yourself (DIY) women feel empowered because they learn their hair while styling and experimenting. Those women who remain dependent on hairdressers or extension styles were often frustrated and overwhelmed because they need to interact with their hair.

The key to embracing this feature is learning to work with tightly coiled hair, not against it. Recondition your mind to understand that length is not a measure of hair health, shrinkage can be deceptive. Your hair texture can present challenges because different sections of the hair can and will react differently when styled. Fortunately, there are ways to work with characteristics of tightly coiled hair like shrinkage and texture. It is a matter off learning your hair's likes and dislikes when styling and using products.

Embracing all the features of tightly coiled hair is part of the journey. For example, when I want to wear box twists, the front of my hair constantly unravels because 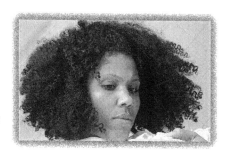 of my loose texture in the front and on the sides. To help it stay together, I might braid in that section or use aloe vera gel for a better hold. Remember, there's no way to change the pattern of tightly coiled hair physically without applying a chemical. By learning how to work with the hair, flexible options can achieve desired results. Take into consideration your varying textures; there really is no short cut.

Understanding why the hair coils is vital. Tightly coiled hair also emerges from the hair follicle in a tight, coiled pattern because of two key traits: the formation and abundance of the water sensitive curl bonds cris-crossed pattern and the shape of the hair follicle. Unlike tightly coiled hair, straight or chemically relaxed hair has parallel bonds. The chemical story is pretty amazing. In the spirit of simplicity, just know that the curly bonds are the key to the spiral formation, because the bonds are the glue that link the hair proteins together forming an alpha helix formation, akin to the shape of DNA or a tornado. Geometrically everything in nature with this formation yields and contains power. That includes tightly coiled hair that may draw up to a length of 1 inch, while stretched to a powerful 10-12 inches!

These bonds as well as the size and shape of the hair follicle, determine the nature of the tightly coiled hair. All life is birthed from this formation because DNA is the foundational blueprint of every living thing, body and cell making everything unique. Because of this awesome relationship between nature and us, these spirals are worth understanding and worth appreciating. There are enough books and websites that separate hair types based upon curl formation. I don't believe in categorizing our hair into letters or numbers. This categorization of hair continues to divide women into different camps. I choose to refrain from using comparisons because through my journey, I found categorizing my hair was counterproductive. The bottom line is tightly coiled hair is a microcosm of many textures.

Another feature of transitioning hair is scab hair. Scab hair is hair that has been damaged from years of relaxing. The coil pattern resists curling and usually lays straight. The solution is to continue trimming until the hair reverts to its coiled pattern when moist. A good test is to spritz hair with water. If it curls, keep your grow on. If it remains straight, trim it away.

Look at the following pictures. I dare you to find a texture like yours. Look for: sheen, shine, loose curls, tightness, tender patterns with sharp bends and turns. Some heads lack curls, ringlets *and* definition, they just simply exist as a bouquet of cotton. Some hairs may

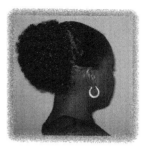

clump together in ringlets, others won't. Some of the ladies have curly hair at the roots and straight hair at the ends. Many have a loose texture up front or at the nape of the head. Others have wiry, coarse hair in the middle of the head. Still others have tightly coiled hair everywhere else. There will be no curl measure chart here. Just know that tightly coiled hair that I refer to is just that: hair that is tightly coiled, shrinks a lot and needs moisture to thrive.

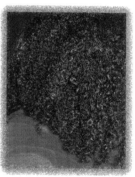

Yes! Our hair grows, the many bends in the strand make length difficult to discern...so take pictures and record your benchmarks of growth and health that the naked eye cannot see. More importantly, the picture will be the inspiration when the journey feels hard and unproductive. Stay flexible and try not to type cast your hair. Just as we are all individuals, so is each strand, section and patch of hair.

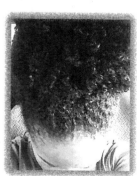

Empowerment allows you and your hair to symbiotically work together, exploring and enhancing the nature of the curl, the beauty of its praise and pattern of its texture. Explore online albums, find what works for different ladies. Find ladies with hair similar to yours and explore what styles, products and maintenance programs work for you.

Both the mental and physical transitions take time, patience and commitment. The reward for waiting, growing and learning is a mind with a mature awareness, self-love and a beautiful head of hair at the end of the journey. This is not for the snicker bar folk who want to slap a track in the head and glue it to hair and have an instantaneous flow of hair. This journey is for those that want steak, slowly cooked, sizzling with taste and a side potato, steaming with butter. This is a journey for folk that have time for self. Those people who know that the investment is worth divestment from a dominating mindset that will never value African features as the standard of beauty. This journey is for the sister who values herself enough to know who she was created to be. It is for the woman who can accept the bend of her curls over the superficial 'ease' of a chemical to straighten the hair to appease another's standard of beauty.

How do you know when the mental or physical journey is over? It's over when it doesn't matter anymore. It's over when you accept that this is who God made you to be. It's over when you demand that others accept that this is who you were born to be, unadulterated and true. The journey is over when you feel complete and unapologetic about your naps in the presence of those lacking them. Then and only then will you be ready for another level, another journey that can take you even further, beyond hair and beyond care.

TRANSITION STEPS

1. *See your Vision* (This step is so important and perhaps the most difficult.) Set realistic and tangible goals, to make the journey easier. Embrace every aspect of your life with pictures that inspire, motivate and encourage you. See yourself in your natural state. Keep a journal of your journey, especially note products and effects on your hair.

2. *Write your Natural Vision* Periodically, write your 'why' and your goals because they may change as they evolve around your vision. Reassess your 'why' to keep you focused on your personal contract. Refer to the resources listed in this book and from the growing cyber community of naturals to build a support network. Reflect on the small steps it will take to help you complete your goal as the vision manifests. Set estimated timelines and benchmarks.

3. *Crown Yourself* Once the goal is met, reward yourself. Go out with your new group of natural friends and celebrate with a Henna Party or a girlfriend's hair party. You've come along way!

Knotty Note

Often women, like me, who choose to go natural are often proud of their heritage. We have accepted our lot in life. Our hair is kinky and we would rather work with it than deny self. When we have a sense of who we were made to be and accept who we are, we take pride in wearing our hair in its natural state.

CHAPTER FOUR

YOUR TRANSITION
hairstyles that get you to the other side

Take the kinks out of your mind, instead of your hair.
-Marcus Garvey

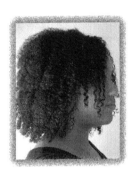

Tightly coiled hair commands attention and nurturing. It is naughty by nature, fragile by design, and strong all at the same time. If the wrong products are applied, or inappropriate tools are used to 'control' it, it will react by tangling. Tangling from split ends, breaking from heat or hair tools, improper or impatient handling or mishandling will occur unless you know what you are doing. The first concept to understand is there will be 2 opposing textures that meet at the line of demarcation. The line of demarcation is where the new virgin hair growth meets the relaxed hair. The line of demarcation is very fragile.

34

RESPECT THE LINE OF DEMARCATION

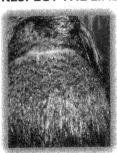

Notice the new growth and the chemically relaxed hair. Where they meet is the line of demarcation.

Because the line of demarcation where the virgin, tightly coiled hair meets the chemically processed hair, avoid tension from hair pins, bands and heavy brushing or combing at all costs! Hair is weakest where the new growth meets the chemically relaxed hair and **even more fragile when it's wet.** The virgin hair is tight, and contracts from moist conditions. The chemically treated hair is fragile at the line of demarcation as the parallel bonds are weakened when they meet the criss-crossed bonds of the virgin hair. The two textures would rather break off ties literally and figuratively than deal with one another. It is important to be caring, nurturing and considerate to this dynamic by working with the natural hair texture, not against it. Massage hair with olive oil two or three times a week to keep it moisturized, healthy and nourished.

Any straight style *will* work against the line of demarcation as the bonds are weakened by the two opposing textures. Curly styles emphasize texture and complement the moisture depleted environment, stabilizing the bonds and protecting your hair. Wet sets with a curling tool of choice or braid outs/twist outs work well. When the hair is wet, add Aloe Vera gel and olive oil to moisturize and set the wave pattern. A cold blow dryer setting is the best option to dry the hair over heat which can damage your transitioning hair.

To reduce breakage at the line of demarcation, never comb your hair straight through from root to end, comb with your fingers first. And, please, please, please never comb or brush wet hair with improper tools. To make it more pliable, spritz your hair with water and a light moisturizer when detangling in sections. Comb it from the ends to just below the line of demarcation with a large tooth comb until it's detangled. Move up the strand to the root, systematically detangling in the same careful order: fingers, large toothed comb or brush. Secure the sections with a terrycloth pony holder, duck billed clip or a china bump if hair is long enough.

35

TRANSITION OPTIONS

Determine which transitioning style works best for you. Don't take the mental part of this journey for granted; your hair is unique. Going natural is so much more than learning the right methods and products to style your hair. Make the transitioning process fit your personality and lifestyle. The journey is manageable, possible and irreplaceable. If you learn to do things yourself, you won't have to fire your hairstylist, you can work with them to learn your grade of hair and how to manage it.

It is important to remain flexible, it may seem easier to chemically relax the hair and submit to the dependant cycle of the hair care industry— but what would you learn about yourself in this journey called life? Aren't options great to have!

TC/ the Transitional Cut

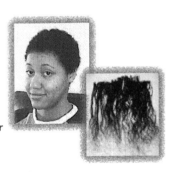

Transition for months then gradually cut off one to two inches a month of processed hair. The transitional cut is a gradual way to grow the chemical relaxer out of the hair as hair is trimmed 1-2 inches per month.

Transition Cut with Braid Extensions /Braid-and-grow-out

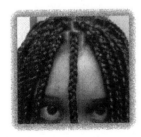

As time progresses, the chemically relaxed hair is trimmed until all that remains is unadulterated hair. By wearing braid extensions or interlocked weave, the hair grows to the desired length chemical free.

Wigs & Hairpieces

Transitioning with hairpieces, falls/half wigs, and wigs can be sassy and fly. It's important to use gentle tools under the hair that won't rip out the hairline or cause breakage. Be careful with those hairlines, making sure the piece isn't pulling on the roots of the hair!

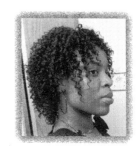

GB/Go Bald

Cut off all your chemically processed hair and start fresh! That's right, like Kojac, shave it down and grow a fresh bouquet of hair. Are you bold enough?!

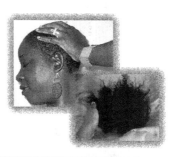

37

Knotty Note

My daddy always loved my little afro and loved over my hair. It was subliminal outside peer pressure that caused me to relax my hair in high school. Just like dating, my mom made me wait until I was sixteen to get a relaxer. I wanted to do the latest styles and it wasn't possible with my cottony hair. At football games in 9th grade, in the night air, my hair swelled into an Afro. I noticed that all of the other chemically processed girl's hair stayed straight during and after the game. I watched in amazement as their well placed heat set curls stayed in place. No one cajoled me into relaxing my hair; the styles around me did. As a teenager, I began to experiment with my hair and demanded chemically relaxed hair, too. But when I got it, all it did was lay flat. It didn't hold a curl. Then it broke off in a vicious cycle until I cut it all out of my head.

MGeorge, 2007

TREAT YOUR BODY RIGHT!

Health in your mind, body and soul is important! Everything from this point on should be about 'feeding' your hair, as it reflects you inside and out. Whatever goes into your body comes out somehow, even if it's junk. From bad skin, unhealthy weight, and digestive problems, your hair also grows with deficiencies if it lacks proper nutrients. If you find your hair dry and need a solution, immediately increase your water intake. Actually, the recommended eight glasses of water a day is the minimal amount!! Try to reach for 60 to 100 ounces, or half your body's weight in water per day! If your body is dehydrated, dandruff will indicate that the scalp is moisture deprived.

Adding fiber to your diet will help the hair, so try eating a bowl of steal cut oatmeal in the morning. This type of oatmeal is usually only found at specialty stores. If steal cut oatmeal is too gritty or chewy for you, fix regular oatmeal, staying away from the packaged, processed stuff which has the least amount of nutrients. Not only will your hair thank you for it, but you may loose a few pounds as well, (an extra bonus)!

It's also important to eat protein from meat, fish, poultry, eggs, nuts and grains to replenish the hair cells with amino acids, rich in nutrients for growth. Go lightly on the meat, thinking in terms of fiber, which is found in whole grain foods, fruits, and vegetables. It's important to eat non-refined carbohydrates from veggies, fruits, whole grains, brown rice and potatoes for energy and hair growth. Eat good fat from nuts and/or fish for shiny hair. Keep junk food to a minimum! Think of hair like a plant and water it! Feed it omega 3 fatty acids, fruits and vegetables. The body does not know how to translate and properly break down processed food with lots of hard to read ingredients. Say no to candy bars, chips,

38

pop, or at least eat them in moderation.

STAY AWAY FROM HEAT!

Remember: *transitioning hair is fragile.* If you compromise
the health of your hair with heat, it can cause
irreplaceable damage. The line of demarcation will
disintegrate even more from the heat. Health of hair can
slowly degrade the cuticle exposing the core, causing
gradual splitting and fraying. If heat is applied to the hair
in the form of hair dryers, blow dryers, curling irons or
other appliances, there will be consequences. A sign of
heat damage is hair fraying and not lying down. When
more heat is applied to smooth the hair, the hair still
isn't crisp, neat, or shiny, it will stay bumpy, crunchy and
unruly—never completely returning to a smooth look until
it is cut out. Trim a strand of hair, examine it and notice
the holes, tears, and splits, sometimes two upon 4, upon
more. There will probably be splits all along the strand
of the hair. Everyone's level of heat resistance varies
and the only way to test out the point of no return is to
apply heat to the hair. If you want to test the affects of
heat upon your hair, test it on shed hair, not hair on your
head.

39

As thick as tightly coiled hair appears, it is the most
fragile of any hair type and it will show the effect of heat
application almost immediately. Nothing can reverse heat
damage except cutting it out! So, unless you're prepared
for a drastic haircut, leave it be. Nothing, I mean nothing
— ACV, conditioning treatments — nothing, will reverse
the damage. So, learn hairstyles that complement tightly
coiled hair, without the heat and the hair will beautifully
flourish. If you do use a blow drier, use a diffuser on a
cool setting. To keep the hair in tip top shape keep it
simple: be gentle, no heat, use water, protect, and use the
right products.

PROTECT THE HAIR AT NIGHT

To preserve the health of your hair, remember to wear a satin bonnet or scarf at night. The scarf will protect the hair from nighttime tossing and turning which can lead to bed head, knots, tangles and damage. First, remove all hair tools before sleeping! Apply moisturizer of choice before lying down to make your tresses happier while you rest. Long, loose natural hair should be spritzed, put into large braids and satin covered. If the hair is not long enough, you can secure hair with a satin scarf. If you are wearing curlers or large twists or braids, a satin bonnet may be more comfortable.

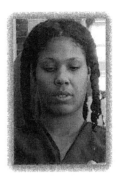

USE GENTLE HAIR TOOLS

Say no to hair tools that create tension, especially elastic ponytail holders and tight headbands. These tools pull on the hair like a small knife that methodically cuts the hair, breaking it into shreds. (Transitioning hair is especially susceptible to this type of damage). Keep hair loose, alternate tools regularly, and make sure they have a protective coating. Be gentle with your temple hair, when hair is stressed, these areas will show signs first and in some cases the damage cannot be reversed, resulting in bald patches.

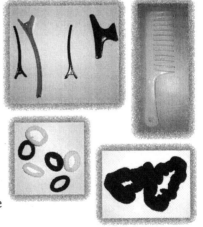

Use wide toothed combs, terry pony tail holders and always keep a spray bottle with conditioner handy. Get creative with your tools! Many have used cut pantyhose, ribbons, socks, belts, bra straps, head bands (loose fitting) and scarves. Just remove the tool at night and replace in the morning if desired. If a curly style is desired, satin covered hair curlers are soft, cushy and make cute curls, while protecting the hair.

Hair buckles, large bobby pins, scrunchies, and spandex material headbands are other great styling tools that help protect tightly coiled hair. An accordion comb secures hair because tension is adjustable; it's a great option when hair is too short to wear in a bun. The hairstyle possibilities with braids, twists and loose hair are endless with the right tools and patience!

Brushes   41
A Denman Brush© (D3/D4) or any wide tooth brush with plastic covering can detangle the hair sufficiently. The Denman Brush© is wide and stiff, making it a pliable tool to remove shed hair without damage. Denman Brushes© can be used on wet hair. When using the Denman Brush©, detangle a section of hair by coating it with a moisturizer and separating the tangles with fingers, if possible. The Denman Brush© is good for detangling, but if used too harshly, like any tool, it can pull the hair out.

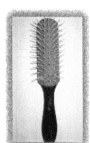

Denman Brush©

Another brush which smoothes hair once it is detangled is a natural bristle boar brush. Boar brushes are critical because synthetic brushes tend to rip out hair and create split ends. Boar brushes are often used to smooth or calm frizzies. A baby brush with a conditioning spritz is

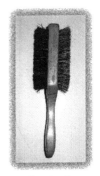
Boar brush

another alternative to prevent breakage and smooth the hair, because of its gentle bristles. Remember to spritz with water if necessary to assist the detangling process. Be gentle and patient as you secure the detangled sections with a duck billed clip, Bantu knot or plait. Like your makeup brushes, hair brushes and combs should be washed after use. Try to clean them at least monthly!

ADDITIONAL HAIR PRODUCTS

It is important to care properly for both textures by infusing plenty of moisture and nutrients. The chemically altered texture needs nutrient replenishment, the proper balance of moisture and the proper balance of proteins. The new growth needs special nutrients and care, but not always in the same amount or form as treated hair. Care needs to be made that the two textures are not stressed from the moisture and tools used for maintenance. The second part of the mind reconditioning is relearning what is healthy for the hair. Products that work well for 'artificial' hair usually don't like natural hair and it shows immediately, the product will sit on the hair and skin, instead of being absorbed. When the chemically free hair does not react at all to a product, record the product, its ingredients and how it was used for future reference.

The secret to growing healthy tightly coiled hair is moisture, proper tools and the right products! Stay away from petroleum, mineral, and silicone based products; they give the user a false perception of conditioning while strangling skin and hair of much needed

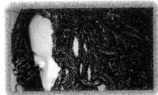

42

moisture, contributing to dry, damaged hair. It appears moisturized because the hair is shiny. Do not be fooled! Derivatives of crude oil used on the human body inhibit oxygen exchange and suffocate the hair. Chemically processed hair does not like these products either. Nevertheless, relaxed hair will behave decently, deceiving you of its ineffectiveness.

Focus on moisture as well as strength and protection. Products that lock in moisture are critical. Once again, beware of products that suffocate the hair: petroleum, mineral oil, lanoline, silicones, and its derivatives are all ingredients to look for and stay away from. They give the user a false perception of conditioning while strangling skin and hair from moisture, contributing to dry damaged hair.

IT'S ALL ABOUT THE PRODUCT

Knotty Note

My focus is on the basics first. Because every product line is not for everyone, there are many product lines and many ingredients to choose from that nourish and condition hair. Far too many to continue using a favorite hair grease that mama and "nem" used to straighten hair!

JUST SAY NO!
There are good products and bad products for your hair. Eliminating the ingredients and products found in the "Just Say No List" on pages 44-46 will be hard, but it is necessary. ***Please become an avid reader of the ingredients list. No more picking up branded items!!!! Choose items with the right stuff!*** Throw out products that are harmful to your body.

THE JUST SAY NO LIST

Ingredient	Where Found	Hamrful Effects	Hair Uses	Linked to Cancer?
PETROLEUM (a derivative of crude oil, cutting oil, and lubricating oil)	Conditioners Moisturizers	Headaches, flushing/skin discoloration and redness, dizziness, mental depression, nausea, vomiting, narcosis, and even coma.	When applied, hair appears shiny and moist, yet it prevents moisture from getting in and out while attracting dust and suffocating hair.	
MINERAL OIL	Conditioners Moisturizers	Headaches, flushing, dizziness, depression, nausea, vomiting, narcosis, and even coma.	Hair appears shiny and moist, but is suffocated.	
PROPYLENE GLYCOL	Food Hair Products Cosmetics Antifreeze Medicine Fake smoke Pen ink Stamp pads De-icing solutions		Pulls water out of hair, drying it out.	Yes

INGREDIENT	WHERE FOUND	HARMFUL EFFECTS	HAIR USES	LINKED TO CANCER?
SILICONE	Products for shine and sheen Breast implants	Ongoing studies to determine health impact.	Makes hair appear shiny and moist, yet moisture is locked out. It creates a wall, preventing other products from penetrating the hair shaft.	Yes
PROTEIN (with caution)	Conditioners Moisturizers	Rinse your hair well because overuse of protein can damage the hair.	Proteins can be a good thing; in this case, protiens should be balanced with moisture for replentishment. Follow the directions precisely! Choose a wheat protein if there's a choice.	
ALUMINUM	Coloring dyes	Aluminum on the hair can lead to breakage from drying out.	Fresh chemical applications can not be coupled with a dye job.	
DEA (Diethanolamine) MEA (Momoethnanolamine) TEA (Triethanolamine)	Personal care products in the form of: Cocamide DEA or MES, Lauramide DEA	Has been proven to transfer from skin to bloodstream quickly and completely; Chemicals disrupt the body's hormones.		Yes

45

Ingredient	Where Found	Harmful Effects	Hair Uses	Linked to Cancer?
Sodium Hydroxide Calcium Hydroxide	Antifreeze Products that clear clogged sewage drains Relaxers	Carcinogenic, burns, irritates, and must be used with caution and protective gloves.	Lye and No Lye perms	
Beeswax	Pomades Hair grease Conditioners	Beeswax suffocates the hair.	Hair shines for a little while, then build up comes with trapped lint, dust, and debris.	
Synthetic Dyes, Perfumes, Coloring, and Additives *(with caution)*	Coloring used in personal care products	All things synthetic are not dangerous. However, all things synthetic are not natural to the body either. Caution is suggested, especially for highly allergic/asthmatic individuals	Animal studies have proven these to be carcinogenic.	Yes
SLS (Sodium Laurel Sulfate) SLES (Sodium Laureth Sufate)	Shampoo	Linked to blindness, diarrhea, skin irritation, death, and is carcinogenic; Is a vehicle of nitrate transmission into the body; Very drying to hair.	Used to create lather in shampoo.	Yes

Once I eliminated these 'do nots' from my routine, my hair began behaving wonderfully. For example, my style of preference was twist outs and as my natural hair grew over two inches, my relaxed hair did not behave. It looked dry, felt sticky and didn't hold a style. At the line of demarcation, my new growth did this funky thing with shrinkage: it coiled and didn't twist. My tightly coiled hair hated pink setting lotion. The relaxed ends twisted nicely with it until the two textures grew to equal lengths. After a while the relaxed ends looked stringy, that's when I decided to cut the relaxer off and used natural products from that point on.

Your hair may do something unique as well. You may have the intention to grow your hair out for 12 months or more. If you get to this point of discontent, as I did, you have reached one of the first pivotal turning points along your journey. You will either move forward and cut the dead, relaxed ends off—or you will turn back and relax your hair. It is my hope that you, the reader, realize that many before you have come to the same crossroads. You too can move forward and press on to win your prize as well: a beautiful crown.

Glycerin is one example of a product on the *Just Say NO List*. It can be found in moisturizers, conditioner and sometimes shampoos. Use glycerin with caution because it adds moisture to hair **when** moisture is in the air. However, in warm climates and dry winter months it will dry out the hair, pulling moisture *from* the hair. The key to glycerin's benefits is that it works best in **moist** climates. Use in the summer to draw moisture from the air for deposit into the hair; leave alone in the winter. Review the following chart for other products and ingredients that are not good for our hair such as formaldehyde which is used to preserve dead bodies but can be found in makeup and hair products.

47

Contrary to the "Just Say No List," here are some lists of "Can Do" products that your hair will love.

CARRIER OILS

To keep tightly coiled hair in its best shape, use moisturizing products such as carrier oils derived from vegetables, nut or seed oils that retain and supply moisture. These oils have therapeutic properties and present a good source of nutrients and energy. They can be in liquid form, or solid (i.e. shea butter, which needs to be emulsified by the palm of the hands).

Through trial and error, find which moisturizer is best for your hair. If your hair does not like a moisturizer, it will bead up and sit like raindrops on a leaf. To test a product, apply a sample to the back of your hand. If your skin absorbs the oil immediately, it usually will work for your hair.

The following liquid oil moisturizers can be used on their own, or with essential oils. Just remember that oils put nutrients in the hair and moisturizers replenish the hair with moisture. Our hair needs both. A combination of 8 oz of oil with 8 drops of essential oil will usually satisfy these requirements. Some plant oils that contain nutrients and in some cases moisturize can be found on the following page.

48

CARRIER OILS

Coconut Oil	Moisturizes and conditions may attract insects, 'bee' careful!
Olive Oil	Economical moisturizer/conditioner.
Almond Oil	Moisturizes and conditions, non-greasy, easily absorbed.
Apricot Kernel Oil	Spreads easily on the skin. Rich in essential fatty acids, oleic and linoleic acid.
Castor Oil	Attracts moisture to the hair. Unlike glycerin, won't dry the hair oil. Penetrates well and will increase elimination of bowels as it seeps into pores. Has dual cleansing powers and cheap!
Avocado Oil	Will infuse vitamins A, E, D and potassium into hair and skin. Additional benefit of protein, so be careful if using another protein product.
Jojoba Oil	Moisturizes and conditions, excellent sebum replacement, a natural cleanser.

49

ESSENTIAL OILS

Never use an essential oil directly on your hair or skin! Always dilute with a carrier oil or water; it is fine to use both. Buy genuine or Grade A to validate its' purity. If you purchase an oil and do not know its authenticity, take notes on how it effects your hair.

All of the essential oils found on the following lists are known for their strong qualities. They offer nutrients, assist hair growth and combat various hair and scalp functions. There is not one that is overall better than the other; each comes with its own specifications and limitations. The one that is best for your hair is the single most important qualifier. Start with a basic one like lemongrass or jasmine and go from there. Take notes with the included charts, so you can remember the results on your hair. An essential oil is used to enhance nutrient replenishment. Add an essential oil to your carrier oil in incremental drops, ie. with 8 oz of carrier oil, use 8 oz of essential oil.

ESSENTIAL OILS

Chamomile	hair sheen, conditions
Basil	hair growth
Peppermint	promotes hair growth
Cedarwood	antiseptic, cleanser, toner; treats dandruff, increases growth
Eucalyptus	cleanser
Frankincense	stimulates sebum production
Lemongrass	clean fresh smell. slows down oil production
Rosemary Oil	aids in hair growth (not for pregnant women)
Tea Tree Oil	treats oily hair, dry scalp; natural antiseptic
Ylang Ylang	antiseptic, stimulates growth; controls sebum production
Lemon	cleanser, hair lightener
Lavender	soothes senses, treats dandruff
Sage	natural cleansing and reviving properties of dead hair follicles

51

MOISTURIZERS

Horsetail	hair growth, protection, collagen stimulation
Shea Butter	moisture, softens, and protects*
Aloe Vera	promotes healing of dry/damaged hair/ skin, moisture
Olive Oil	moisture, softens, and protects
Vitamin E	protection, hair growth
Almond Oil	moisture, sheen
Coconut Oil	moisture, sheen
Jojoba	cleanser, conditioner, moisture, softener
Honey	cleanser, moisturizer*
MSM	strengthen and soften
Vegetable Glycerin	lubricant, soften, moisture, protection*
Pantheon	moisture, protection, sheen, hydration
Biotin	body, shine, hair growth
Cholesterol	emulsifier, lubricant**

*moisturizers that may be in solid form
**is a protein, so be careful

When combining ingredients pick an oil base for the foundation, such as olive oil or one of the other oils mentioned on page 49. It can be purchased from the local food club and used sparingly throughout the whole year, because a gallon of it lasts for half of a year! You can create individual portions, eight ounces each, for a daily moisturizer. Add a few drops of essential oils to your carrier oil. For twenty bucks, nothing could be better for all of those benefits!

Add one essential oil for a month and see how successful this regimen is for you. Never overload your hair with too many products at one time. If it doesn't work, try another one. Results will be difficult to discern if the hair is not given enough time to react with washings, styling and application.

I rotate between two essential oils, lemongrass (I love, love, love the smell!) and rosemary. Rosemary will stimulate the hair follicles, assisting in hair growth that I've witnessed for myself. However, all essential oils come with their specific warnings and cautions. Rosemary should not be used by epileptics or pregnant women; it may cause a miscarriage.

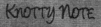

Knotty Note

An example of a simple daily spritz:
8 oz of water or Aloe Vera juice in a spray bottle
Add 8 drops of rosemary oil
8 drops of lemongrass oil and
1 teaspoon/5 ml jojoba or olive oil
Spritz enough to feel a tingle. Hair should not be damp,
just wet at the touch.

Rub a quarter-sized amount into your palm and evenly distribute throughout the head from root to end. By adding the essential oils, more nutrients will infuse into the scalp and hair. The internet is a great resource to research the oils, indications and contraindications.

In the winter, or all year 'round, water can be replaced with Aloe Vera juice (found at the health food store). Aloe Vera juice provides extra nutrient rich ingredients that feed the hair, which is an advantage during the arid winter months. Once again, the whole purpose is about moisture and nutrient replenishment, giving the hair what it needs from the inside and out. It's important to play around with various carrier oils, finding the one that compliments maintenance routine and hair. I choose to stay away from 'sweet' oils like coconut; others have reported how the scent causes summertime bees to chase them. I also know of people whose scalp has reacted badly to olive oil. The critical factor is to know personal preferences and options. Raid somebody's pantry (mama or a friend) and get a week's sample of a plant-based oil to try.

MOISTURE AND HOLD

Aloe Vera gel is a great natural product for hold; it locks in moisture as well as defines curls. For holistic reasons, some people stay away from preservatives. I have used Lilly of the Valley©, which is purchased at the health food store and Fruit of the Earth© found at Wal-Mart. Lilly of the Valley© must be kept refrigerated. Aloe Vera gel is an excellent holding agent that can help 'pop' curly waves bringing definition to the spiral curls of tightly coiled

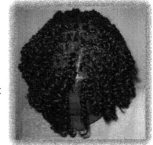

hair. It works without drying your hair because it infuses moisture and nutrients, while locking it in.

Other natural products for hold, nutrients and definition are: castor oil, honey, flaxseed, coconut oil, and glycerin (Preferably use glycerin during the summer and spring, as it draws moisture from the air into your hair. If used in the winter, it will pull moisture from the hair, evaporating into the air). Once again, add a quarter-sized amount into palms, rub together and apply to the hair and scalp.

The moisturizing regimen can be kept simple with a personal house mixture with natural ingredients that you can purchase. Keep it simple with plant-based carrier oils with essential oils and a moisturizing holding agent like Aloe Vera gel. There are many product lines that can be purchased at salons/stores or online. I do not endorse one over another. I do have my preferences, simply because of my personal experience. If a product line you are interested in is not mentioned in Addendum IV, read the ingredients for safety and try it, making notes! Any omission on my part is not reflective of the quality or reputation of a company, it is simply personal experience.

55

Each and every strand of hair is unique, so assuming that one product has the same effect on every head is not going to happen. Presently, there is not a hard and fast formula that will work for all hair types and variations. Please use the product suggestions as a foundation to build upon and tweak for personal use. To prevent product junky disease (PJ), the ingredients I suggest are basic for a good foundation. The books and websites listed in the resources will lead you on many wonderful adventures and places to spend your money. If your funds are limited, keep it simple and stick to the basics; three alternate products should work. You can add or substitute later, just keep good notes!

More simple conditioning spritzes and solutions can be found in Mireille Liong-A-Kong's book <u>Going Natural: How to Fall in Love with Nappy Hair</u>. In addition, the resource section includes web resources that can further assist you on your search. Take this book with you to the store, read the ingredients, do your homework and begin the process!

HAIR RULES
1. Respect the line of demarcation!

2. Use the techniques and styles to complement your transitioning hair.

3. Focus on healthy hair and body not LONG hair.

4. Do not use heat; water is your friend.

5. Protect your hair at night.

6. Use gentle hair tools; never comb or brush dry hair. Always spritz it with a light solution that incorporates moisturizer.

7. Read your hair product labels!

Five / Clean Hair is Happy Hair

CHAPTER FIVE

Clean Hair is Happy Hair
Washing and Conditioning

Before we all went synthetic, before chemicals, before hot combs, Grandma used natural products and they worked for a good reason! The Bible mentions the use of hemp, olive oil, figs, hyssop, flaxseed and the like. Starting with this foundation, with our tools

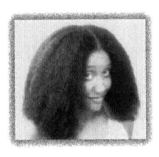

and products in place, is a good place to begin for good reason.

58

SHAMPOO TIME
The first step to perform when shampooing the hair is a manicure. That's right, a manicure. Trimming and filing the cuticles and nails prevent unwanted snagging, tugging, pulling, and damage to the hair. Whenever I do anything to my hair, ideally, I will inspect my primary tools, my hands. Make sure to smooth, cut and trim away cuticles, protruding skin and jagged nails.

Shampooing the hair is a straight forward process with a few critical steps. When tightly coiled hair is washed, it can be a simple, pain-free event if you follow the steps. If one step is avoided, the hair can mat and tear from tangled knots that may not easily come undone. Ninety percent of the battle is knowing how to manage your tightly coiled hair. These steps are: **conditioning, sectioning, detangling, shampooing with a plant-based**

shampoo, rinsing, condition (again) and **detangling**. This process is also known as CSDSRCD. Is CSDSRCD really necessary? YES, YES AND YES! Let me explain why.

Conditioning
It is best to **condition** the hair with olive oil (or any conditioner) over night or 30 minutes before shampooing first in preparation for any tangles in the hair prior to manipulation. One way I ease the battle is by preconditioning with olive oil or a cheap conditioner the night before. I cover with a shower cap and secure with a scarf to help the hair strands wash with reduced tangling and increased pliability, moisture and shine. Thirty minutes minimum is good, overnight is best. Less time would only waste a good conditioner, while doing nothing for your hair.

Sectioning

Hair banding is the process of securing a section of hair with a terry coated pony holder. The benefits of banding are to stretch the hair, reduce frizzies and keep hair tangle free. Coils and baby locks can be washed with banding. Box braids or twists can be washed by banding and loose hair stays less tangled via banding. If a section of hair is banded and secured with a pony holder, it will prevent the hair from unraveling and tangling.

Another example of banding is prepping a large section of

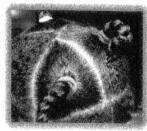

hair to shampoo it as shown in the picture. The section can be washed inside the band. With the pads of the fingers, lather under the hair at the scalp. To wash the hair, squeeze until the water turns clear. If banding is used on dry hair, it may stretch the hair out, combating shrinkage. Another benefit to banding is to stretch and lengthen a hair style as it dries. A great technique to counteract shrinkage.

Detangling

Detangle hair with a large toothed comb, Denman Brush© or your fingers. Gently comb through each section from ends of hair to the root. Once the section is detangled, band it until you're ready to shampoo. This is very, very important. Unlike straight hair that combs from scalp to ends, tightly coiled hair must detangle upwardly from end to roots first to minimize knots, tangles and matting. There's nothing worse than a mass of matted hair in the middle of the head to contend with from lack of detangling during the wash session.

Shampooing

There is a debate in the Internet community, which evolves around using or not using SLS (Sodium Lauryl Sulfate) or SLES (Sodium Laureth Sulfate, the alcohol form of SLS). SLS is the ingredient that creates soap bubbles. SLES is slightly less irritating than SLS, but may have more drying properties. On their own, SLS and SLES are not dangerous; however, they have the ability to act as a catalyst to cancer by assisting in the formation of nitrate and dioxin formations. Ironically, this is the same ingredient found in car wash soaps, garage floor cleaners and engine degreasers. SLES/SLS are just one of many chemicals our body encounters on a daily basis from toothpastes and cosmetics to engine degreasers. With this potential risk and the drying affects of shampoos, it's preferable that you implement plant-based shampoos that are user friendly and safer for you and the environment.

I prefer plant-based shampoo because they have the ability to clean and hydrate with plenty of moisture.

Look for shampoos based from either olive oil, rosemary, peppermint, Brazil nut, wheat proteins, fruit and plant extracts, sunflower or coconuts. The shampoo does not have to have all the ingredients; this is just a sampling of the *type* of ingredients to look for when you shop. A bar of African Black Soap can also be used to wash and moisturize the hair. Work up a lather in the palm of your hands. Then, lather it into the hair and work it into the scalp then squeeze the soap bubbles through the hair, using it like a regular shampoo. When using any shampoo, it should be diluted and used sparingly.

HOW TO SHAMPOO
Prep your shampoo by diluting 1 capful of shampoo with 8 oz of water in a spray bottle. Spray sections, work up a lather, squeeze the hair and massage ONLY the scalp with finger pads. Try to reduce manipulation of the hair as much as possible. Tightly coiled hair is at its most fragile when wet and prone to breakage. Make sure to wash in a sink with a good spray attachment. Continue to wash each section. Rinse with the hair in sections. Rinse the soap out by gently squeezing out the water like a sponge, until all the section is free of soap residue. For a visual go to *YouTube* (www.youtube.com) and plug in terms such as: washing hair, curly hair, etc.

Rinsing
It's important to **rinse** to get rid of the soap and product residue after shampooing. A rinse is usually done with a mixture of apple cider vinegar and water, affectionately called an ACV rinse. You need a spray bottle, baking soda, apple cider vinegar (ACV) and water. Add a pinch of baking soda to your spray bottle. Then, add 1/8 cup ACV to 3/4 cup water in the spray bottle. Mix gently because the baking soda and ACV will react and try to bubble over. Spray hair section-by-section, working through massaging, squeezing and pumping. Let it sit

61

on the hair, while you complete all sections. Protect your eyes for the mixture may sting. Rinse thoroughly by squeezing and pumping until the water runs clear.

The purpose of the ACV rinse is to clean the hair of product buildup and balance the PH. ACV can help to seal the hair cuticle and provide slippage to assist with detangling. ACV rinse is a nice option, when there's a need to remove build up when hair is dull and lifeless. The ACV rinse will help rid the detergent residue, returning the hair back to a neutral PH state. The ACV rinse does not have to be done every time; however, it can be done for extra cleaning, leaving the hair soft, manageable, and most importantly, clean!

Conditioning
Condition your hair in sections; finger comb or use a wide tooth comb to keep hair in a detangled state. If you choose heat, sit under the dryer to open the cuticle for 20-30 minutes wearing a plastic cap. If you prefer to avoid heat, purchase a 'heat cap' (it looks like a gold shower cap). Place a towel on top of the cap for 15-30 minutes to seal in heat and moisture. Rinse until the cold water is clear and free of bubbles. Make sure to rinse with the cold water to help seal in the benefits of the conditioner. Apply a leave in conditioner, such as olive oil while that section is tangle free, then band with a terry pony holder.

Detangling
And, of course, after conditioning, please **detangle** again so the hair can be styled with the least amount of drama. Once hair is detangled thoroughly, secure in braids or twists until time to style.

At all times, tightly coiled hair will get along better if the coils are separated as much as possible. The coils like to hang in cliques, tighter than glue. If the coils dry that way, then they are harder to separate. After hair is blotted dry, apply a quarter-sized amount of olive oil to the palm of the hands, work through and massage into a section of the hair at a time. An alcohol free gel or Aloe Vera gel can be used as well, for hold and definition. Once the plaits are in, air-drying the hair is preferable. If not possible, sit under a bonnet dryer or put two or three scarves on and call it a night. Wake up and your hair may be dry. If it's not, damp hair is the best to manipulate anyway, so proceed.

You can also dry your hair with the special micro fiber towels that can be purchased at your local drugstore. Rubbing hair with a regular towel can damage the hair by creating more mats, tangles and knots. Luckily, microfiber towels hold a lot of water! The motion to dry should be the motion you used to squeeze water through your hair. Squeeze and pat to dry the hair. Forget about the sexy commercials that show the woman with long flowing hair whipping it back, rubbing a towel through her locks and smiling into the sunset. By now, we know that tightly coiled hair 'don't do that!'

It's been proven and true that CSDSRCD works. The process may be called different things; but, the end result is the same: clean, tangle free hair. If tightly coiled hair is washed like the ladies in the commercial who wash and rinse in one sitting you will PAY for it! An incredible amount of time will be spent detangling matted knots of your hair. Just think of the benefit of strong, buff arms because of caring for your tightly coiled hair. Remember, all hair, chemically treated or natural, thrives when the proper ingredients are used. Let's face it—going natural is not for everyone. Using natural products can be.

63

THE ART OF CONDITIONING

When looking for a good conditioner, focus on hydration from plant based products as well. Ingredients that tightly coiled hair love are Aloe Vera gel, wheat germ, hemp, olive oil, shea, nut and other naturally occurring plant materials that seal in moisture. Choose a simple product, such as olive oil. With this simple ingredient, you can't go wrong. There's a tendency, for naturals to become product junkies. The hair thrives best when ingredients are streamlined and simple. I stick with an olive oil based shampoo and for my conditioner I use olive oil tweaked with a few drops of lemongrass for scalp nutrition and aroma, that's it! Hair will grow happier and healthier than ever when a simple regimen is chosen and adhered to.

Knotty Note

A nice pretreatment for hard, brittle hair in need of intense attention is a hot oil treatment of olive oil. In the microwave, warm a cup of olive oil. If you can touch the olive oil without getting burned, yet it's warm, that's perfect. Coat your hair section by section until scalp and hair are saturated with olive oil. Squeeze out excess and cover with a plastic cap. Let it penetrate the hair for a minimum of 30 minutes. Move onto the shampoo phase.

When conditioning tightly coiled hair, focus on moisture retention. Become educated on products that seal in moisture and do the research, become empowered, read labels, research the ingredients. It's good to use the most natural, purified version of a moisturizing product. Be careful, these products can get rather pricey and the same results can often be met with a more cost-effective option. Some simple, important ingredients (although there are others) to look for in conditioners can be found below.

CONDITIONERS

Shea Butter	moisture, softens, and protects
Aloe Vera	promotes healing of dry/damaged hair/skin, moisture
Olive Oil	moisture, softens, and protects
Vitamin E	protection, hair growth
Almond Oil	moisture, sheen
Coconut Oil	moisture, sheen
Jojoba	cleanser, conditioner, moisture, softener
Honey	cleanser, moisturizer
MSM	strengthen and soften
Vegetable Glycerin	lubricant, soften, moisture, protection
Pantheon	moisture, protection, sheen, hydration
Biotin	body, shine, hair growth
Cholesterol	emulsifier, lubricant

65

Second to moisture is protein. Protein can strengthen the hair strand by strand by incorporating amino acids temporarily into the hair shaft making the strand stronger. My use of protein conditioners has been limited due to the fact that in my experience, my tightly coiled hair stiffens then it snaps and breaks easily if I use the wrong amount of protein. Once the hair strand becomes fortified with a protein conditioner, it can be prone to breakage. Therefore, a good combination of moisture and protein is necessary for pliability as well as strength. Pay special attention to the directions on a product with protein. Too long on the hair could lead to breakage down the line. Protein treatments come in the form of amino acids, animal or wheat. Animal protein can be harsh, wheat is usually more forgiving. Once again, test and try. Read all ingredients and keep notes of what is used, how it is used and the results.

66

Knotty Note

How to tell if you need more moisture or protein:

1. If you stretch your hair and it stretches A LOT, then practically stretches apart, barely snapping at all...your hair is in need of protein.

2. If your hair doesn't stretch and snaps weakly, crumbling away in a tight ball, it needs more moisture. If pulling causes the hair strand to break, it needs more moisture.

CO-WASHING

Co-washing is a term used to describe washing the hair with conditioner instead of shampoo. Dilute a capful of conditioner in a spray bottle and then wash each section as you would with regular shampoo. Some experience extreme dryness from regular shampoos and prefer this method, because conditioners have cleansing ability as well. Others, like me, cannot co-wash. My hair does not like it. I found if I simply dilute my shampoo in a spray bottle with water, by adding 1 capful of plant based shampoo to eight ounces of water, my hair thrives. The co-wash leaves my hair heavy, and my scalp retains a film of product and dirt that I just could not eliminate with simple conditioner. The only way to find out if this method works is to try it a few times.

Some of the reasons to co-wash are:

- Hair needs more moisture during winter months

- Swimming hair needs more moisture from chlorine

- Work out hair may need a co-wash to replace a regular wash because frequent washings dry the hair

- A co-wash may complement a wash-n-go style: co-wash, pat dry, shake, then go!

CHAPTER SIX

DIY: Do It Yourself Trims
How To Cut and Maintain Your Hair:
If You Want To That Is!

Tightly curled hair *can* grow long — only if you keep it trimmed. Keeping hair trimmed is important to promote growth healthy growth! The foundation to a head of healthy hair is proper maintenance inside and out, topped off with a good trim. This chapter will explore advantages and disadvantages to hair trims at home, or at the shop.

Naturally curly hair is prone to dryness which causes splits that can run down the length of the hair strand. It can be a mixture of wiry texture with sharp to loose bends, wavy texture, sharp coarse texture or straight texture! There are so many variations that can exist on one head. The bottom line is it is important to stay on top of trims because tightly coiled hair is fragile. It looks tough, full, and thick; however, it has fewer cuticle layers than any other hair type, which offers less protection from heat, wear and tear. Less protection also means it is easily damaged. Someone with wavy, straight hair may be able to use a blow dryer without damage because they have more cuticle layers. Someone with tightly coiled hair can easily damage the hair if heat is applied, because of the thin cuticle layer.

There are quite a few factors that affect the moisture level of tightly coiled hair. This texture produces a lot of sebum, the protective oil that coats the hair strand. However, the sebum does not reach the full length of the hair stand, without brushing the hair, preventing lubrication of the hair: another reason brushing is important because it helps to distribute the sebum along the hair shaft. As a result, the strands can become coarse. Strands may begin to have tiny knots along the length of the strand. Eventually, the knots will turn into tears and splits, which will lead to damage. Because this hair texture winds upon itself, it can form split ends from simply getting longer. Splits are formed when the cuticle is compromised and the cortex splits at the ends. With manipulation and time, the cuticle continues to split from the ends to the root like a pealed banana, exposing the cortex's vital nutrients. With length, comes more turns, coils, and eventually splits. Since tightly coiled hair is prone to damage from nature, manipulation, tension, heat and stress can further magnify the problem. If heat is applied to hair, hair is stripped of moisture, the seal is cracked and splits will occur.

Once the seal of one fiber along the strand is opened, that strand will continue to split towards the root/scalp and must be cut off to stop from splitting further. If your tightly coiled hair is prone to damage, trimming the ends monthly (a method referred to as 'dusting') may be best. Dusting is a micro-trim that can keep the hair looking healthy and strong. The stronger the strand, the less it will result in premature damage from split ends while growing.

For example, I dusted my loose natural hair. My hair growth was not compromised because my hair grows about a half of an inch per month. I literally would just snip the ends off about quarter to an eight of an inch. Since I dusted on a monthly basis, I never missed the length.

DIY VERSUS PROFESSIONAL TRIM

To some, there is nothing better than being in charge of his/her own schedule and hair maintenance. There is confidence, restored time, and flexibility in becoming a DIYer. DIY trimming results in self-confidence because you have no one else to blame! Another advantage to DIY is heat aversion. Many stylists find it a challenge to trim naturally curly hair unless it is straightened. Because heat can damage hair, I would prefer to have a trim with wet hair or dry, 'stretched' hair. I always sought a happy medium: healthy natural hair that was trimmed without the damage from heat application.

Think about it, the coil pattern sets in, shrinkage sets in, and style sets in all while relinquishing control to the curl. The straight lines that come with chemically straightened hair are not important with a head full of curls. What is important is the *shape* of the hair—that's it! Embracing the form of the hair, allowing it to take form and grow into a natural shape that frames the face is enough. Letting go of straight lines is one of the healthiest things you can do for yourself and your pocketbook! If your hair is straightened, most tightly coiled naturals will attest that the hair stays straight for a maximum of 3-5 days, between the humidity, sweat and life, the curl pattern takes over once again and the benefit of pressing is quickly lost. To extend the life of a style, DIY trims are easy, flexible, cheap and effective because you are doing it yourself.

The obvious reason to get hair trimmed professionally is to get a straight cut, especially at the back of the head. For this reason, just as many natural heads opt for a professional cut. If this is your preference, pay attention to the amount of heat applied to the hair, the length of time the heat is applied, and the heat protectant used. Request that the stylist add a moisturizing protectant to the hair first and minimize the heat application to a medium setting on the blow drier before trimming. Some stylists may try to add additional heat for straightening with a flat iron. JUST SAY NO.

The price of 'temporary' straightening is not worth the damage the heat can do to the curl pattern of the hair. A reasonable option is a cold blow out, when the hair is blow dried or set on a cool setting. A cold blowout can also be plaiting the hair in 4 large sections and allowing the hair to air dry.

Heat can alter the texture of the coil pattern, giving the hair a loose, fragile curl pattern. When this occurs, only growing it out can bring back the curl pattern, because the protective cuticle has been damaged. The protective cuticle *will* crack from the heat, so protect yourself and request a protective sealant and a low to medium heat setting when your hair must be blow dried.

Finally, understanding the anatomy of a hair strand is also important. Because each hair strand is made up of three parts: the medulla, cortex and cuticle, it is critical to protect the hair strand's fragile framework. The medulla is the center pulp area, which contains melanin. Melanin determines hair color. The cortex is the protein layer that contains proteins one of which is keratin, and many other amino acids and nutrients. Keratin is the protein in the hair that gives the hair strand its strength. The cuticle is the protective outer coating of dead cells. When the cuticle is compromised from stress, it cracks leading to a split end. Now let's get to cutting!

Whether choosing DIY or professional, consider how the benefits and disadvantages effect daily maintenance:

Do you mind paying someone to trim your hair?
Do you like to be pampered?
Do you mind being at the mercy of someone else's schedule?
Do you like to style your own hair?

KnOTTY NOTE

How do you know it is time to trim?

You know it's time for a trim if . . .
your hair feels dry, like straw
your ends feel crunchy, are frayed or look bad!
your hair is extremely frizzy
your hair tangles more than usual, as if glue were holding the strands together
you haven't had one in 12 weeks

The more tightly coiled the hair, the more likely frequent trims are needed. Trimming every month is a method called dusting, allows you to stay on top of the damage either right when it occurs or before the hair is compromised. Dusting is a process that eliminates damaged ends with frequent, monthly trims of less than a quarter of an inch of hair. When chemically relaxing, the hairstylist usually trims the hair on a 10-12 week rotation, by a quarter to half of an inch. Learn the appropriate time to trim your hair; pay attention to its needs and what it responds to. Read the signs: damaged hair begins showing sings of dullness, frizziness, breakage, and hair loss.

On my own hair, I have seen the splits occur above or below the knot, or in both directions. I have seen holes through strands of hair that look like the eye of a needle. I have seen strands of hair that double, triple and quadruple split up the shaft of the hair. Then, knots can occur at the base of the hair strand or any other point. If left alone, the damage will lead to severe shedding. There are many creative ways to trim, loose hair can be cut in sections, twisted or braided hair can be cut in sections as well. By conducting an internet search, it's easy to find a method that fits your style. Let's explore!

Knotty Note

DIY is not for everyone. I learned through trial and error:

1. I can trim my hair and like the results.
2. Tightly coiled hair does not need to be cut even.
3. Tightly coiled hair by nature can have varying textures. When I DIY, I can treat each section individually. Just as every nappy head is different, every hair on a head thrives when treated uniquely.
4. All I need is a good pair of scissors, a mirror, clips, my hands and moisturizer.
5. When I made a mistake it was only temporary, my hair grew back! I would have been angry had it been someone else who jacked up my hair!

LET'S DIY!
Have all of your supplies laid out and ready to use:

1. Manicured Hands

2. Scissors

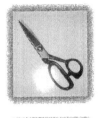

3. Mirror

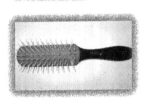

74

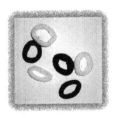

4. Brush

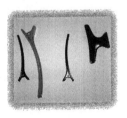

5. Coated Pony Holders

6. Duck Billed Clips

WAYS TO TRIM

Always remember that you want to start with a clean head of hair; damp hair is best. Make sure that your supplies are close, laid out and ready for use before you start. If it is still too difficult to cut evenly, go to a hairstylist and allow them to trim your crown. The back will be difficult, but remember with time and practice, it can be accomplished. It's important to deprogram yourself from expecting straight ends with a straight cut. For four months try one method of trimming. In addition, choose your times between trims: monthly, 12-week trim or 6-week trim.

PART-IT-TRIM

Parting the hair in sections is an easy way to trim the hair. This method is ideal for dry, straight *or* wet, curly hair. This trim will give the hair *shape* not straight lines. The cut will usually lead to a layered look as well. For those who prefer healthy hair over even hair.

75

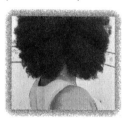

1. With a large toothed comb, separate hair into two large sections.

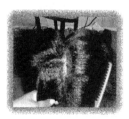

2. Continue to make sections.

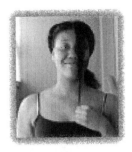

3. Secure each the sections by braiding, banding, and clipping with duck billed clips).

4. Brush each section as straight as possible, pulling away from the head.

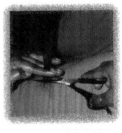

5. Examine the ends paying careful attention to the dips and peaks.

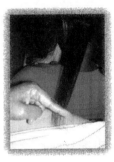

6. Trim the dips and peaks away, cutting away all the split ends, valleys and peaks so there's nothing but an even line of hair left.

7. Secure the trimmed section and move on to the next.

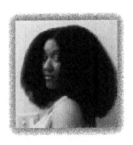

8. Continue the pattern: secure, trim, secure trim. Repeat for all quadrants. If a large section is too big to work with, just make smaller sections within the section to trim and secure until the quadrant is complete. The result will be a layered, shaped hairstyle.

TWO-STRAND TWIST TRIM

This method is also ideal for straight and curly naturals who prefer healthy hair over even hair. It can be done on dry hair or wet hair. The look will usually lead to a layered look as well.

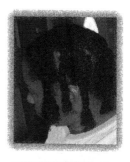

1. Partition hair into large sections.

2. Split each section. The size, shape and amount of the twist will vary.

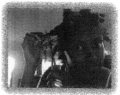

3. At the bottom of the twist, section hair between index and middle finger. Snip off hair where the ends are uneven.

4. Retwist and move onto the next twist.

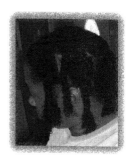

5. After snipping ends, add a light moisturizer of choice, paying special attention to the ends. Good job!

BLOW IT OUT (HEAT, DRY HAIR) TRIM

This method is ideal for curly naturals who desire straight ends that complement a particular hairstyle. I do not add heat for a temporary style because it can leave permanent damage. Heat is very damaging for tightly coiled hair. When the hair is exposed to heat, the cuticle can break exposing the strands to split from the central core strand. In some cases, the detection is immediate. If time and preference are a factor, blow drying may be for you. Remember, be careful if you choose to blow dry, use a cool setting. You can also section your hair into large plaits or braids to air dry.

1. Part hair into sections.

2. Secure each of the four sections with a coated pony holder or duck billed clip. Brush each section as straight as possible. Gather section and pull away from the head.

3. Split each section and secure.

4. Blow out the section, secure and rotate until the whole head is dry. If drying in the hood dryer or air drying, wait until the head is completely dry.

5. Brush and stretch the hair away from the head, trim eliminating the peaks, and valleys at the tips of the hair.

6. Secure trimmed hair and start a new section.

7. Apply a light moisturizer to the ends when complete. Lina, a member of Fotki provides a solution for an excellent protectant at okorolina40@hotmail.com read more about this on:
    http://www.growafrohairlong.com

To minimize damage, minimize the following practices:

1. Just say NO, NO NO to heat!
2. If you color your hair use natural products, such as Henna, that minimize moisture depletion.
3. Reduce the use of styling tools, or at least alternate. Your hair can suffer damage if exposed to too much of any hair tool.
4. Coat collars, hats, wigs or other clothing: Can cause friction, resulting in damage to the hair.
5. Rotate between at least three hairstyles to reduce damage or leave hair in one protective styles for 2-3 weeks.
6. Be proactive — think protectively. When hair is not able to freely move (bound in a plait, braid or twist without accessories) it is 'protected' from the elements and styling tools, allowed to rest and grow.
7. Moisturize the ends daily.
8. Find styles that incorporate moisture and complement the curly pattern.
9. Trim naturally curly hair every 4-10 weeks.
10. Invest in a good pair of scissors!
11. Wear a protective satin cap under your hat!

CHAPTER SEVEN

GETTING YOUR HAIR DID

When we are liberated from our own fear,
our presence automatically liberates others.
-Marianne Williamson

Many women have chosen to document their journeys online because of their passion for natural hair. Most journals can be found by posting a search on www.fotki.com, www.blogspot.com, www.picturetrail.com and many other online photo journals. Because my research began on www.nappturality.com, this is where my picture search began. As a member, you have access to photos, journals, tips and experiences. It is because of my shared experience on nappturality.com that this chapter can be brought to you. Because of my own shame of going natural in corporate Amerika, I did not document my hairstyle experiments, failures and successes.

80

At one time I was both ashamed of and determined about my napps, I am now determined to further the cause. I share their stories because in the course of writing this book, I have travelled along another path—the path to locks. It is a new, and very different journey that has involved a deeper level of focused concentration. Because I don't want to confuse the two separate journeys, I trust that my sisters will give you vision of the beauty of your tresses. My journey to lockdom has taken me to another level that I intend to share in another book. For now, enjoy the many beautiful styles you can create with your loose, natural hair. I thank my virtual sisters who have kindly provided their photos to help me. We hope that by seeing these beautiful sisters and sharing in their journey, you will see the endless possibilities of the beauty that lies under the lye. DO YOU and LOVE YOU.

The style chart below will help you understand your hair-style options for various stages.

STYLE CHART
NATURAL & TRANSITIONING HAIR STYLE CHART

Type of Style	Protected Hair (PH)	Chemical Free Hair (CFH)	Transitioning Hair (TH)
	These styles promote growth, reduce damage, and limit hair maintenance to a maximum of once per week. Style can be left in the hair for two months if desired.	*Styles for chemical free hair only.*	*Your two textures of unprocessed new growth and chemically relaxed hair can agree.*
Afro		X	
Afro Puffs*	X	X	X
Bantu Knots	X	X	
Braid Out		X	X
Buns*	X	X	X
Curls	X	X	X
Extension Hair	X	X	X
French Rolls	X	X	X
Kinky Twists	X	X	X
Micro Braids	X	X	X
Plaits	X	X	X
Shake 'N Go		X	
Straw Set	X	X	X
Twists	X	X	X
Wraps	X	X	X

* Buns and afro puffs gently pulled back and covered with a hair piece can be protective.

TWISTS AND TURNS

Box braids and twists allow for a lot of flexibility. Sizes can be super tiny and micro or super thick and massive. The advantage of small braids or twists are the multiple style options, washable hair (when banded), and low daily maintenance. Keep in mind, the smaller the sections, the longer it will take to finish and remove! Styles vary from updo French rolls to buns, twist outs, braid outs, cornrows, and roller sets.

HOW TO

1. Prep hair with conditioning spritz spray.

2. Make four large sections and secure with pony holders.

3. Section hair as desired for boxes of plaits or braids. Braid or twist to the end.

4. Section off a centimeter or more area of hair the size of a pencil eraser top.

5. When large section complete, secure with a duck billed clip or pony holder. Move to the next section.

For hold and curl definition, use Aloe Vera gel or castor oil. Hair butters, such as shea butter, can be used as well. At night, tie sections in bands to keep hair stretched, with more length. Massage a

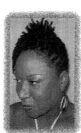
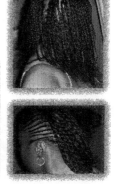

Lots of braids and twists of all shapes and sizes. There's plenty of flexibility and fun without tangles and knots.

light moisturizer and a satin scarf to secure. If flat in the morning, lightly spritz and finger tussle to plump and define. For extra curl, set on rollers and secure with a satin bonnet at night. Have fun! Every 2-3 days apply a moisturizer from the "Can Do list" that your hair likes. Experimenting with wet hair, dry hair, setting lotions, butters and oils will also offer various options and looks. This style can be left in for up to two months. A nice benefit is that your hair can still be washed with the braids and twists in it as long as it's banded! Again, be careful and take braids out after two months with a good moisturizer or it will result in locked hair.

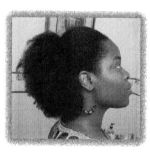

AFRO PUFFS
Afro puffs are cute, but be careful and persistent with dusting/trims if you wear this style frequently, to stimulate healthy hair. The safest way to wear the puff is with the ends are tucked away from the elements under a bun. When wearing an afro puff, keep moisture in mind, and limit the style to one or two days a week at the most! Tension from the bun holder, pulling hairline and fragile ends can take a toll on the health of the hair. Remember that the tension can be reduced by implementing the accordion comb which can SAVE THE HAIRLINE. Refer back to the chapter on gentle hair tools for new ideas. At night, wear a satin scarf to preserve your hairstyle and remove all tools. Spritz in the morning and repeat the smoothing process for another clean afro puff or bun.

HOW TO
1. Prep hair with conditioning spritz spray, then tease the hair into position with fingers and a boar head brush.

2. Secure as much hair as possible with a large scrunchi (if hair is in locks, twists or braids move to step 7).

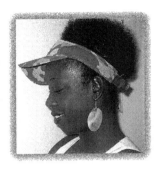

3. If hair is loose, smooth with Aloe Vera gel and brush until smooth.

4. Secure with the scarf or scrunchi, adjusting tension accordingly.

5. If you don't have enough hair to place in a true bun there are options:

    a. Cover the pony holder with a black headband, scrunchi or scarf

    b. Leave the pony holder exposed

    c. Add synthetic kinky hair to the bun or a natural ponytail extension for fullness. Secure with bobby pins if necessary.

    d. Take off the scrunchi and reapply over the accordion comb. If you used bobby pins, be sure to cover them with the scrunchi around the bun, neatly tucking the pins.

6. Secure hair and smooth with more Aloe Vera gel if needed.

7. Place a satin scarf on smooth part of hair for 15 minutes to set the style. Now, go and be fly.

THE BUN

Buns are a polished way to present natural hair in a corporate environment, at the beach, or on the street. You can make buns with braids, twists, loose, or added on hair. Use headbands, scarves, texture and add on pieces to spice it up! If the hair is going to be kept loose in an afro puff, keep a spray of your favorite spritz mixture on hand for some mid-afternoon refreshment — those ends can get thirsty and dry.

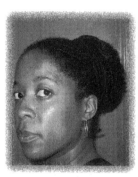

Buns are considered protective if there is no tension on the temple hair, and a smooth hair holder such as an accordion comb is used in lieu of a pony holder. In addition, if your hair is secured under a fake pony tail and tucked, not loose and curly as in the afro puff style, it also protects your hair. To protect ends, covering the massive afro puff with a curly piece that complements the hair texture is an option. For further protection, some women sware by this technique: simply slather a moisturizing conditioner onto your ends, wrap them in a plastic baggie with a fake pony tail. They claim this technique can reduce knots, tangles and matting, while protecting the hair. I have tried it and it does work. You be the judge. Just know that there are options out there for you!

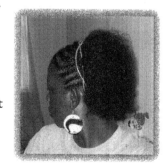

PLAITS

Plaits are braids or twists that are attached along the scalp and do not hang loose like boxed braids. Plaits can be

85

done with boxed twists and loose braids the same way! You can leave them in for up to 2 months without hair locking and matting. It's important not to braid/twist too tightly. If small, white bumps are felt or seen, after installation: STOP! It's too tight! (If you are using a stylist, take control and communicate so the braid can be redone right away). Undo or redo any taught sections. It WILL lead to traction alopecia. Be sure to leave plenty of give for a comfortable hairstyle.

HOW TO
1. Spritz hair with conditioner.

2. Section the hair accordingly.

3. Secure loose hair away from the section to plait/twist.

4. Within sections, separate into three pieces for braids and two for twists. Braid/twist while picking up hair until the end of the parted section is reached.

5. Style as desired.

6. Keep conditioned with moisturizer every two to three days.

7. Secure with a satin scarf at night.

8. Spray a conditioning moisturizer for ease of removal.

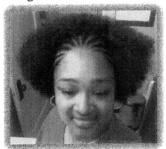

Use large plaits or twists as solutions to counter bed head which is the condition of hair tangling and matting when sleeping. Get creative with your plaited braids and leave a section out for a dramatic effect. They are also perfect to secure hair after washing. Sit under the hair dryer to obtain a chunky fro look. Experiment and find what is right for your look! Whichever style you choose, seriously consider the size of the braids/plaits. Remember, braids take more time to put in *and* take out!

CURLS AND MO' CURLS

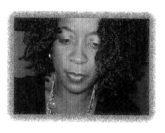

Curls come in many sizes and styles, that's what's so nice about them! Curls are as versatile as you want them to be. Curls can be done with box braids, twists, loose hair, transitioning hair or locks.

Your curls can be as tight Shirley Temple curls (created with straws or rods) or as loose as a flip. Experiment and see what works best for you. Remember to finger comb your curls – only!

For all the time, patience and work rollers take, I always found that a good braid/twist out yielded comparable results. If curls are

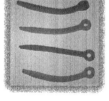

your desire, play around with different rollers, briadouts, or twistouts to get the look you desire! I have also used straws, U- shaped rollers, paper bag ties and pipe cleaners. The time you choose to invest and the desired look is the primary

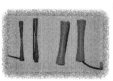

consideration. Once the curls are set under a hood or bonnet dryer, maintain by gently rubbing in a light moisturizer such as olive oil every two or three days, sleep with a satin bonnet and tighten up loose curls with some setting lotion and a roller or two over night to refresh the look. Have fun!

HOW TO

1. If hair is dry, spritz lightly for a quicker set, or set by parting and rolling sections after washing.

2. Apply holding gel or setting lotion to the section of the curl. Secure with an end paper and set the roller. Sit under dryer to set curls. There's nothing worse than taking out the curlers without a curl.

WRAP IT UP

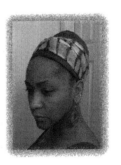

Headwraps can be convenient when you want to be stylish on a bad hair day. Long scarves can be wrapped around the head and secured by tucking the ends under; or to partially cover your hair as well. You can wrap your whole head with something as simple as a T-shirt. Wraps give style and punch to your look, protection from the elements and give a discreet way to dry your hair while you run around with the kids (I do it!).

HOW TO

(taken from fotki member CongoBrava, visit http://public.fotki.com/CongoBrava/locd-life/loc-styles/headwraps to see more headwrap ideas and tutorials)

1. Pick a t-shirt, any t-shirt will do as long as it can cover your head and wrap fully.

2. Turn the t-shirt up side down so that you're holding the bottom.

3.

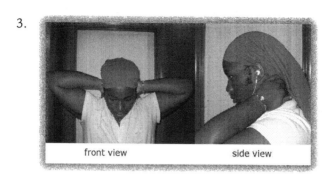

front view   side view

Place the bottom of the tee (thats now in your hands) on top your head like shown on the left. then grab at the ends like shown on the right.

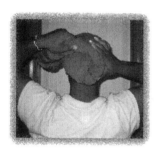

4. Wrap the extra cloth around your head like you would for any other wrap.

89

5. Tuck it in and VOILA!

Note: if you have a lot of hair, it might be best to put your hair into a ponytail or bun prior to doing this headwrap.

SHAKE-N-GO/WASH-N-GO

The key to the wash-n-go is finding the product that works for you. It should contain a moisturizer than can hold and retain water, help the sheen in your hair to come out and give the desired curl definition.

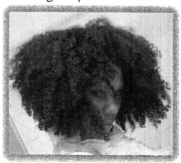

HOW TO

1. Wash and condition your hair.

2. Apply a product from the "Can Do list" with fingers. DO NOT COMB OR BRUSH THE HAIR WITH ANYTHING EXCEPT YOUR FINGERS!

3. Wrap your hair with a micro fiber water absorbent towel for 10-15 minutes: plopping.

4. Take off the towel.

5. Shake your head and go!

HOW TO PLOP FOR A WASH-N-GO STYLE
Plopping

Plopping is the process of wringing out wet hair after it is washed without manipulation. No detangling, no combing, no brushing. Just wash, place the microfiber towel on the hair for 10-15 minutes. For curl definition, sheen and moisture, some women prefer to massage a hair dressing (such as Aloe Vera gel with olive oil) and conditioner for extra moisture after plopping. Plopping is often associated with the hairstyle called a wash and go. Plop when you are short on time and want a healthy alternative without the hours of detangling and styling.

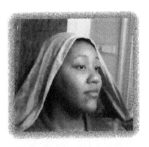

1. Fresh out the water, with a "Can Do" moisturizer, massaging into hair with fingers only, turn head upside down and wrap a towel on top of head.

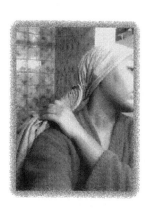

2. Twist towel on head by making and X formation.

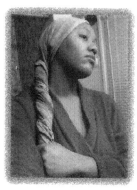

3. Cross and twists ends of the towel around one another.

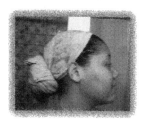

4. Secure and let dry for 15-20 minutes.

AFRO

Afros are everywhere! Moisture is the main concern for afro wearers. Finding a good moisturizer that lasts all day can be challenging and critical. Carrying a spray bottle of your favorite spritz concoction will be the life saver you need to sport this fly hair style. Hair exposed to the elements (sun, wind, rain and heat), has a tendency to

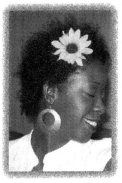

dry out quickly. Wearing the afro with texture (i.e. knots, knot outs, twist outs, braid outs, etc) seems to help retain moisture better than picking it out. In addition, when you have been exposed to the elements, coat your hair with a conditioner, cover with a plastic cap and satin scarf for extra replenishment and protection at home overnight.

It takes confidence and poise to rock an afro. The nice thing about the 'fro is that you cannot get bored with the look. You are only limited by your own imagination and length. Don't let shrinkage fool ya! With 2-4 inches, the possibilities grow even more. Let's explore the afro:

Take a fro and...

- put a headband, scarf, bow or flower in it
- chunk it up with Afro knots or Bantu twirls
- do a straw set
- twist/twirl it in sections during the night and let it out during the day
- put in twists, either comb or finger (achieve finger twists by pinching hair with your thumb and index finger)

- pick it out, plait it up, let it out
- put braids, plaits, twists or afro knots at the hairline
- create small coils

KINKY TWISTS, MICROBRAIDS, EXTENSION HAIR

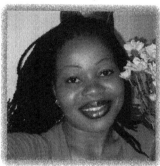

Transitioning with braids or kinky twists is quite controversial. Many have successfully done it with the key focus on care and moisture. Keep in mind, once you are completely natural, extensions are still an option because they can give a much needed rest to the hair and your hands! The extensions should not be installed tightly under any circumstances.

If you get a facelift because the braids are so tight, or they pull your eyeballs up into your hairline, they're too tight. If you see bumps along the hairline, that turn white, the hair is too tight. Too tight hair is a no, no! Absolutely, undoubtedly, redo the braid or twist if it is too tight. If you are paying someone to install them; and, they are installing them tightly, don't pay them until they re-do. You will live to regret it, if you don't stick up for yourself.

Remember to feed your hair with moisture and treat it with care. Use gentle tools: no tight pony tails, no heat, and no alcohol-based products. They may lead to permanent traction alopecia. Frequently,

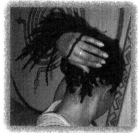

93

use moisturizer and water to keep the hair healthy and refreshed. Be careful, too much conditioning can lead to slippage. A technique to prevent your hair from puffing up through the synthetic hair is to use Organics Lock and Twist Gel™. Smooth it down and cover the hair with a satin scarf at night. The human hair should blend in well with your hair and any daily moisturizer.

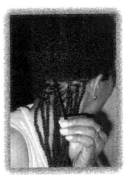

For more information on braiding extensions into hair, see http://www.growafrohairlong.com/. The site allows you to download instructions onto your computer; there's even a video option!

BANTU KNOTS
Bantu knots are fun variations of large sections.

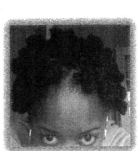

HOW TO
1. Spritz the hair with your conditioning spray.

2. Part first section with fingers or a large toothed comb.

3. Secure the rest of the hair away from the section.

4. Detangle with large tooth comb, fingers or Denman brush.

5. Apply a "Can Do" moisturizing gel to section, such as Aloe Vera gel.

The Knotty Truth

6. Begin turning detangled hair counter clockwise, until hair begins to twist and rotate.

7. Pinch the center of the strand into a U-shape

8. Twirl around the base of the "U."

9. Pin with small, coated bobby pins or tuck under so the hair appears in a small knotted ball (*some secure with rubber bands for hold, I don't like the damage from the bands).

10. Continue until entire head is finished.

If you can sleep with these in your head, wear a satin scarf to protect it at night. Spritzing may upset the neatness of the look, so when you're tired of this look, just let out the knot and let your hair hang down. Remember to finger comb-only!

CARE FOR BRAID/TWIST/KNOTS OUTS
*"HOW TO" IN PLAIT SECTION

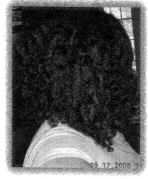

Follow the same instructions for plaits and let the braids/ twists stay in for at least 3-5 days. The longer they stay, the more defined the pattern will be when unleashed. It is critical that only fingers are used to style this look. Any brush, spritz or comb will create frizzies. A light moisturize will keep tresses conditioned every 2-3 days. Sleeping with a bonnet will keep the hairstyle. Be prepared, this style will only last for 2 or 3 days at the most. Hair is more prone to tangling, so be especially careful and diligent when detangling. For years, this was my hairstyle of preference. Because it works with the natural bend of my hair, I only received a chemical relaxer touch up 3 or 4 times a year. When I transitioned out of the chemical relaxer, I used this hairstyle as well. Once natural, it was a perfect addition to my many options.

FRENCH ROLLS

Use hair pins, and spritz to mold the hair into the style of your choice. Remember to take out hair tools at night! Natural can be bold, daring, classy, professional, and stylish! French rolls work well for loose hair and hair sectioned in braids, twists or locks.

HOW TO

1. Brush hair to the back.

2. Gather hair, twist and pin.

3. Begin rolling the hair upwards, pinning every inch.

4. Tuck away the pins.

5. Play with the hair to leave curls or a bang to frame the face.

Whether long or short, the natural hair options are almost endless. The key is your lifestyle and time! Almost anything you did with chemically relaxed hair can be done with chemical-free hair; these hairstyles compliment chemical free hair and transitioning hair. The references listed (including the websites) are additional wonderful resources for creative hairstyles and instructions. This journey can go as far and deep as you choose. The key is to get on the path that leads you to a freedom that expresses who you really are: au napptural!

KNOTTY NOTE

"...that which is the natural curve of my hips, my lips,
my color and bend of my hair is taboo on me.
On me, it's called ugly.
On them, an enhancement..."

-MGeorge

98

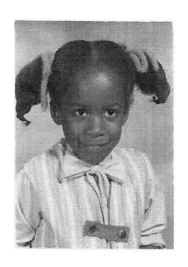

RESOURCES AND REFERENCES

QUICK SOLUTIONS
TO COMMON PROBLEMS

Help! I don't know how to style my natural hair!

Rest assured there are many styles. To name a few: twists, twist outs, box braids, afro puffs (AP), teeny weeny afro (TWA), comb coils, plaits, plait outs and on and on. This book is a hair care manual. Please see Chapter 9 for sample styles. The resources page will also direct you to books and online photo albums and websites.

Help! I don't know how often to wash my hair!

Frequent washing is fine as long as you use products free of SLS/SLES and moisturizer.

Help! I can't find a hat that fits my head anymore. What should I do?

Burlington Coat Factory carries a scarf with give for the head. They are perfect for keeping everything above the neck warm! Other stores carry knitted hats with a brim. Knit has a lot of room for big hair! Caps with give can also be found on etsy.com and other internet sites. Until your length comes, experiment with scarves, ear warmers and head band warmers! There are options for all seasons. When hair hangs from 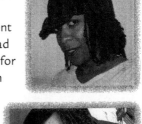 plaits or twists, it will work with a hat!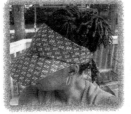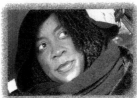

HELP! In the wintertime, I'm worried about damage to my hair as I wear hats and scarves.

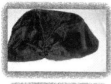

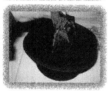

Purchase satin turban hats from a beauty supply store. Either Velcro it into the hat, or just slip it over your hair before your hat. Just tuck it under the hat to avoid detection! You can be fashionable without sporting your bedtime doo-rag out of the house!

Help! My hair is shedding!
Your hair is in a constant state of growth, replenishment and shedding. Preventing rough, split ends can keep hair healthy and reduce shedding. Remember to be gentle and constantly detangle your hair. A good moisturizer and reduced manipulation should help. If problem does not resolve, see a dermatologist that specializes in scalp disorders.

101

Help! I woke up and my hair was matted and won't style correctly!
- Massage a moisturizer through hair and band it or plait it before bedtime.
- Keep a small plastic spritz bottle (4-8oz) of Aloe Vera juice, an essential oil of choice, and a capful of olive oil to freshen hair in the morning.
- Tie hair and secure with a satin scarf.
- Style with hands!

Help! My hair is dry!
Use water, shea butter or Aloe Vera gel. Each product will result in a different outcome, use one product at a time and keep copious notes to remember effects. Protect the

hair with a satin bonnet when in the house. Try to abstain from 'out' hairstyles for at least 3 weeks. Covering the head or wearing in plaits, twists or some other protective style that avoids daily manipulation is a must during those winter months. Stay away from products with glycerin in the wintertime. Glycerin takes moisture from the air. Because of little moisture in the winter, glycerin will do the opposite, and take moisture from your hair.

Help! My hair is in knots and tangles.
Coat hair in conditioner, section, and detangle from ends to roots with fingers or a wide tooth comb. Exercise patience or you will rip knots out of your head. Anytime hair is ripped, the damage must be cut.

Help: My hair won't stay pulled back into a style!
- Spritz hair and smooth with fingers/boar brush.

- Apply Aloe Vera, massage and smooth with fingers/boar
    brush.
- Finish with olive oil to shine.
- Wear a scarf for at least 15 minutes on smoothed hair to set.

Help! My hair is breaking and thinning at the temples!
- First evaluate your hairstyles. Are they putting stress and tension on the hair?
- Use fingers not brush or comb at the edges.
- Tie with a scarf after smoothing with fingers to prevent frizzy edges (do not brush).
- Don't brush at your temples, smooth with fingers, set with scarf only.
- Leave pony tail styles alone for a while; let your hair fall loose.
- Change the tension or type of the pony holder. A cut panty hose is a great option because it's an automatic

scrunchi and the tension can be adjusted.

- Spritz nightly with Aloe Vera juice (8oz) with 8 drops of your favorite essential oils.

Help! My edges have thinned from years of micro braids/relaxers and so has the crown/middle of my head. What should I do?

Find a low maintenance hairstyle and avoid manipulation as much as possible; adapt a protected hair style (see Chapter 7). If necessary, trim away the damage. If you are considering cover up options such as wigs, protect the edges. Keep hair plaited underneath. Spritz the hair with a solution of Aloe Vera juice every other day. To help stimulate hair growth, wash and plait hair once a week.

Help! My teeny weeny afro is dry!

Coat the hair with (non protein) conditioner at night. Put on a plastic cap and secure with a scarf. Your hair will be soft and moist the next day.

Help! My scalp is itching/sore!

Sometimes shampoo with SLS/SLES increases scalp tenderness and itching. The problem is easily solved when you remove these products from your regimen. Use an (ACV) rinse to jump start and neutralize your scalp. You can compliment with a soothing jojoba massage.

It may also take a while for your scalp to stop hurting after you relax your hair. Chemical relaxers can deaden nerve endings causing damage to your follicles. When your scalp regenerates it may feel tender. Lavender oil and jojoba can nurture your scalp back to health. Tylenol helps with pain and an ACV rinse can cleanse your scalp of any product build up. If this does not help, see a dermatologist.

GLOSSARY

This glossary identifies crucial terms as they are used in this manual.

ACV: Apple Cider Vinegar, a rinse to clarify the hair from residual product. It dissolves fatty acids and regulates PH on the hair.

ACCORDIAN COMB: Hair comb set in a cricle; will hold hair back; perfect to hold afro puffs with at least two inches of hair.

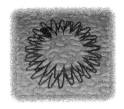

AIR DRY: To let hair dry naturally without applying heat.

AFRO: A hairstyle of tight curls in a full evenly rounded shape.

AFRO PUFF: An afro pulled back into a loose pony tail.

ALPHA HELIX: Shape of DNA, double stranded helix formation, shape of bedspring, formation of tightly coiled hair. Pattern that retains power, energy and force .

BABY BRUSH: Hairbrush made for babies. If used from ends to scalp with a detangler or conditioner, it will gently detangle, hair, reducing knots.

BAGGIE TECHNIQUE: Securing hair in a pony tail, coating ends of the hair with conditioner, sealing with saran wrap or a plastic covering (i.e. shower cap, sandwich bag), to protect the ends.

BANDS: Terry cloth covered pony-tail holders.

BANDING: Process of taking a section of hair and securing with a coated pony holder. The pony holder is wrapped several times around the length of the section.

BANTU KNOTS: Hair is parted and twisted into firm knots and secured to create a hairstyle.

BC/ BIG CHOP/ BIG CUT: Cutting off all chemically treated hair and left with only natural hair.

BLOW DRY/BLOW OUT: To dry hair using a blow dryer.

BOBSA: Black Owned Beauty Supply Association. Birthed to empower women of color and keep money within the black community. Established for African American and Black owned beauty supply stores nationally and internationally. Advocates for Black institutions that depend on beauty supply stores and distribution networks for support to operate competitive hair care services for the black community.

BRAID: A style formed when three or more strands of hair are interwoven.

BRAIDOUT: A style formed when braids are removed from hair and the pattern is set into a wavy appearance.

BREAKAGE: Hair loss due to hair breaking off.

CARRIER OIL: Oil used to blend with an essential oil.

CHEMICAL DEPENDENCY: Relaxed hair needs to have a fresh chemical application reapplied to keep the tightly coiled hair texture straight.

CHEMICAL RELAXER: A chemical hair straightener such as Sodium Hydroxide that changes the pattern of curly hair to straight hair. Must frequently reapply to new growth.

CHINA BUMPS: See Bantu Knots. Hair is parted and twisted into firm knots and secured.

COLD BLOW OUT: Hair that is allowed to air dry naturally and banded to loosen the curl.

COMB COILS: A hairstyle achieved when small comb is used to form coils in the hair.

CONDITIONER: Product that softens and moisturizes hair.

CO-WASHING: Condition wash/no-poo. Washing hair with diluted conditioner and water in a spray bottle.

CORNROW: A hairstyle in which hair is divided into sections which are braided flat to the scalp.

CORTEX: The center of the hair strand.

CNAPP: Someone with napps that feel like cotton. May resemble fine coils, may not because there's no defining pattern.

CREAMY CRACK: Another name for chemical relaxer. Born from the need to constantly retreat hair with chemical relaxer touchups.

CUTICLE: The outer protective later of the hair.

DENMAN BRUSH: Brush used for detangling hair. D3/D4 best to use on tightly coiled hair.

DETANGLER: Penetrates hair shaft to reconstruct, strengthen, soften, condition, and balance pH.

DILUTE: To diminish the strength by mixing with another solution.

DIY: (Do It Yourself); Doing your hair yourself.

DUCK BILLED CLIP: Long clip used to secure hair.

DUSTING: Trimming the hair a quarter of an inch to an eight of an inch every month.

ESSENTIAL OIL/ EO: A class of volatile oils that give plants characteristic odors and are used especially in perfumes and flavorings, and for aromatherapy.

FLAT TWIST: Hair is divided into sections which are twisted flat to the scalp.

FRO: A hairstyle of tight curls in a full evenly rounded shape.

GB: Cutting all of the chemically relaxed hair off, shaving down to the scalp.

GRADE A: The highest therapeutic rating given to an essential oil.

HAIR DRYER: An appliance that dries hair.

HAIR KNOT: When the hair twists and turns into a knot along the hair strand.

HAIR POMADE: Usually a petroleum or mineral based hair dressing for pressing the hair.

HENNA: A chemical free, temporary hair color; a plant that grows in warm, dry climates imparting a red stain. The leaves are dried and ground, mixed with slightly acidic water (and any other ingredients, such as coffee, tea, paprika, honey, etc.), and applied to damp, detangled hair. While most people use it as a safe and healthy way to color hair, it has been used in North Africa and India for many years to make hair long, strong, lustrous, and generally healthy.

HIF/ HAND IN FRO DISEASE: When you can't stop touching your natural hair (mostly because it's soft).

HOT COMB: A steel comb that is heated on a hot plate. Used to straighten hair.

INSTANT CONDITIONER: A leave in conditioner that works upon application.

JOJOBA: A shrub or small tree of Southwestern Northern America with edible seeds that yield a valuable liquid wax knon to have cleansing and restorative abilities.

KINK(s): Tightly coiled hair that rolls into a tight ball, and appears as knots. Can be a general term referring to a head full of tightly coiled hair.

LINE OF DEMARCATION: The border where the natural hair meets the chemically relaxed hair; very fragile and prone to breakage.

LYE/LIQUID DRANO: Chemical relaxer. Lye: synonym for lie denoting the representation that relaxing hair leads tightly coiled hair into a false state of freedom.

MEDULLA: The center core of the hair strand.

MICROBRAIDS: When human hair is braided onto hair creating very small braids of which the ends can hang loose.

MOISTURE: An agent that hydrates. Examples: aloe vera gel, emu oil, jojoba oil.

NAPPY: Hairy or downy resembling the texture of wool.

NAPPY HEADED HO: Term quoted by Don Imus referring to women on the Rutgers Women's Basketball team, (white and black) and their seemingly unattractive appearance and kinky hair. Term highly rejected by those with tightly coiled hair.

NAPPTURAL/NATURAL: A person with hair that has not been chemically treated.

NEW GROWTH: The amount of natural hair grown in since your last relaxer.

PART: The line where the hair is divided into sections.

PART-IT-TRIM: When hair is parted and sectioned to trim; usually secured by bands or clips.

PHAT: A slang phrase meaning something really nice.

PLAITS: Braids, three sections intertwined to form a pattern, usually attached along the scalp.

PONY/PONYTAIL: A hairstyle achieved when a section or all of the hair is pulled back and secured.

PRESS(ING): To straighten hair using a heated implement (usually a specially designed comb).

PJ: A product junkie is a person that buys a lot of hair products.

RELAPSE: Reapplying a chemical relaxer to the hair, after committing to going natural.

RELAXED: Hair treated with a relaxer.

RELAXER: A product used to chemically loosen the curl pattern in hair permanently.

RELAXING: Treating hair with a relaxer.

RINGLETS: Coiled hair bunched together in a spiral formation

ROLLERSET: A hairstyle achieved when sections of hair are wrapped around any cylindrical object and take on the shape of the object.

SCAB HAIR: Hair that grows from damaged follicles. Follicles damaged from years of chemical relaxer application which alters the shape of the follicle, resulting in a change of hair pattern. Observed when natural hair will not curl and feels brittle. Usually subsides within the first year after the last chemical application.

SCARRING ALOPECIA: Hair has been damaged by chemicals that have seeped into the hair follicle causing inflammation, scarring, puss and other reactions. It may result in permanent or temporary hair loss.

SCRUNCHI: A large pony tail holder, usually in a protective cloth material.

SEBUM: Secretion of the sebaceous hair and skin glands, waterproofs and lubricates; protective sealant.

SHRINKAGE: The difference between the actual length of hair and its reduced length after moisture sets in.

SPRITZ: Soft mist of a liquid solution.

STRETCH: Hair that is banded or braided, meant to relax the curl.

SYNTHETIC HAIR: Man-made fibers produced to resemble human hair.

TC/TRANSITION TRIM: Allows hair to grow out of the chemical relaxer; trimming away relaxed hair slowly as new growth emerges.

TEXTURE: The visual or tactile surface characteristics and appearance of hair; basic scheme or structure

TCH/ TIGHTLY COILED HAIR: Hair that spirals into hair coils with the texture of cotton and wool.

TEMPORARY STRAIGHTENER: Used to temporarily alter hair texture (i.e., the hot comb).

TOUCH-UP: Re-treating the hair with a chemical relaxer as new growth emerges from the scalp.

TRACTION ALOPECIA: Hair loss (baldness) cause by friction or pulling.

TRANSITION: Term used to describe journey from relaxed hair to natural hair.

TWA: Abbreviation for Teeny Weeny Afro.

TWIST: A style formed when two strands of hair are wrapped around each other.

TWISTOUT: A hairstyle achieved by twisting the hair and then undoing the twists (often worn as an additional style after two stranded twists).

WHITE PASTE: Another name for a chemical relaxer.

YAK: A form of synthetic hair used for braid extensions and hair weaves.

YARN: A continuous strand composed of either natural or man-made fibers or filaments and used in weaving and knitting to form cloth.

YARN BRAIDS/YARN LOCKS: A hairstyle achieved when yarn is braided onto hair.

113

HELPFUL WEBSITES

www.theknottytruth.com
A website that supports information contained in The Knotty Truth.

www.HealingHerbs.i8.com
A Source of healthy natural ingredients to care for hair. No harsh chemicals or preservatives.

www.nappturality.com
Designed by Patricia Gaines. Members (of which there are currently 67,000), can start threads, post photos, share information, and ask questions pertaining to natural hair.

www.naturallyyoumagazine.com
Founded in 2003, NY! Is the first print magazine to focus on Black natural hair care. Publisher Kaya Casper started it in response to a lack of natural styles and information found in other black hair care magazines.

www.fotki.com
Online photo album that displays personal journals, videos, links and other useful networking tools.

www.picturetrail.com
Online photo album.

locksblogsphotos.blogspot.com
The locked hair blog exchange is excellent for natural hair care ideas. Members post pictures and express thoughts.

www.motowngirl.com
One of the best sites to get a boatload of information on the care of natural hair.

www.bobsaone.org
Website that advocates black institutions that depend

on beauty supply stores and their distribution networks for support, making hair care services for the black community competitive.

www.hennaforhair.com
Site where you can order henna for coloring the hair.

www.naani.com
Site that explores hair options and products for sale.

www.softspikecurlers.com
These curlers are relatively soft and comfortable for sleeping; Ellen will call you back if you have questions.

www.afroworld.com
Buy hair and beauty products.

www.growafrohairlong.com
Black hair care and product website; learn how to grow hair with long braids.

www.going-natural.com
Another spin-off from Nappturality.com. Maesosa offers a magazine, contests, tips and a book on going natural.

www.tytecurl.com
TyteCurl is about the management, empowerment and education of natural hair which has not been chemically treated. They are a group of young vibrant people who wish to encourage our community to love their virgin hair. All the information on the site is put together by their members and freelance writers, who are sharing their experiences as being a part of the TyteCurl global community.

Other natural product lines from sisters at Nappturality. com: Oyin (**www. oyinhandmade.com**) and Asha's (**www. myashas.com**).

A Shopping List

Who Are You?	List 1 Name Brand Diva	List 2 High Maintenance Diva	List 3 Down to Earth, Dolla' Conscious Diva
Shampoo *good options with the right ingredients*	Black Earth Products™ Shampoo	Aveda Brilliant™ Shampoo	Dr. Bronner's™ Baby Mild Organic Liquid Soap; a bar of African Black Soap
Shampoo Options	Burt's Bee Line	Black Earth Products™ Total Body Shampoo	Oyin Line, Asha Line, Sistas Place, Anita Grant
Moisture	Black Earth Products™ Enhancing Conditioner	Aveda Brilliant™ Conditioner	Olive Oil
Moisture Option 2 *recombine if necessary*	Shea Butter	Coconut Oil	Shea Butter
Hold *other options in Chapter 6*	Black Earth Products™ Lock It Up	Aveda Brilliant™ Texturizing Gel	Aloe Vera Gel

Who Are You?	List 1 Name Brand Diva**	List 2 High Maintenance Diva**	List 3 Down to Earth, Dolla' Conscious Diva
Hold Option 2 *see Chapter 6*	Castor Oil	Glycerine (only if humid conditions persist)	Flaxseed Oil
Clarifier *recipe in Chapter 7*	Black Earth Products™ Stimulating Herbal Cleanser	Apple Cider Vinegar, Baking Soda, Distilled Water	Apple Cider Vinegar, Baking Soda, Distilled Water
Spritz *recipe in Chapter 6*	Black Earth Products™ Protective Bodifier	Aveda Brilliant™ Damage Control	Aloe Vera Juice
Essential Oil *(can add to shampoo or conditioner)* *choose from list in Chapter 6*	Chamomile	Chamomile	Chamomile (I prefer Rosemary; pay attention to the warnings!)
Hold Option 2 *see Chapter 6*	Castor Oil	Glycerine (only if humid conditions persist)	Flaxseed Oil

**please read ingredients, some ingredients may not be 100% natural. ALLways read all ingredients in any product!

Product Usage Journal

Make copies of these pages to start your own journal!

Date:

Products Used:

Carrier Oil:

Essential Oil:

Shampoo:

Conditioner:

Moisturizer:

Results:

Product Usage Journal

Make copies of these pages to start your own journal!

DATE:

PRODUCTS USED:

CARRIER OIL:

ESSENTIAL OIL:

SHAMPOO:

CONDITIONER:

MOISTURIZER:

RESULTS:

BIBLIOGRAPHY

Byrd, Ayana D. and Tharps, Lori L. (2001): <u>Hair Story:
Untangling the Roots of Black Hair in America.</u> St.
Martins Griffin, Inc.

DaCosta, Diane with Renfro, Paula T. (2004). <u>Textured
Tresses: The Ultimate Guide to Maintaining and Styling Natural Hair.</u> 2004. Simon and Schuster, Inc.

Herbert P. Goodheart, MD (May, 1999). Hair and Scalp
Disorders P#: <u>Traumatic Alopecia in African-Ameri-
can Women.</u> Women's Health in Primary Care. Vol2
No5.

Keymah, T'Keyah, Crystal (2002). <u>Natural Woman/
Natural Hair: A Hair Journey.</u> T'Keyah Keymah, Inc.

Kinard, Tulani (1997). <u>No Lye! The African-American
Woman's Guide to Natural Hair Care.</u> St. Martins
Press.

Liong-A-Kong, Mireille (2004). <u>Going Natural: How to
Fall in Love with Nappy Hair.</u> Sabi Wiri, Inc.

About the Author

Known to her sistren as
Cheleski (*Shell-ski*), Myra
Michele George lives in
Columbus, Ohio. She shares her
life with her husband and best
friend, Pastor Ronald A. George
and their two sons, Joshua
and Jordan. A graduate with
a BA in Biology from Hampton
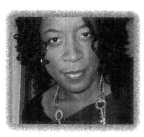
University and a Masters of Science in Physiology from
Clemson University, Chele is a researcher working now as
a Pharmaceutical Sales Representative. On the side she is
a personal trainer, lay counselor and a nappturologist.

Chele's paternal Grandmother introduced her to the
world of beauty. From that beauty, Chele has always
been drawn to the beauty and design of naturally curly
hair. Because *Grandma Gin'* ran a beauty shop out of her
basement, she relayed her passion for hair to "Cheli"
(as *Grandma Gin'* called her) who now manifests this gift
by empowering women to embrace the unique beauty
in their God-made naps. The study, design and art of
natural hair are passions that called Cheli from the
belly of her soul. She has made it her quest to empower
knowledge through teaching others how to love, learn
and care for their own hair. She believes there is ministry
in our tresses and "I have been called to testify." The Knotty
Truth is Chele's first book of many which will enlighten,
educate, and inspire others to live on purpose by
embracing their birth right, rejecting the negative stigma
that has been assigned to our hybrid coils.

122

Women like me, who choose to go natural are often proud of their heritage. We have accepted our lot in life. Our hair is kinky and we would rather work with it than deny self. When we have a sense of who we were made to be and accept who we are, we take pride in wearing our hair in its natural state.

-MGeorge

Made in the USA
Lexington, KY
22 April 2011